POWER
of
POSITIVITY

Coloring Book

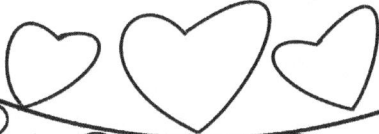

Illustrated
by
Sannel Larson

Power of Positivity Coloring Book

ISBN-13: 978-1543270082
ISBN-10: 1543270085

A NOTE FROM THE ARTIST...

Welcome to the Power of Positivity Coloring Book!
All throughout this inspiring coloring book you'll find
over 30 original hand drawn illustrations that are sure to
offer calm and stress-relieving joy for artists of all ages.

All the illustrations are single-sided so you don't have to
worry about ruining a design on the opposite page.
However, I would suggest placing a piece of paper or two
under the page you are coloring, or a piece of a
cardstock, and the illustration beneath will be fully
protected, so go ahead and use markers, colored pencils,
fine point markers, crayons and pastels.

Thank you to everyone for purchasing my coloring book.
These hand-drawn illustrations were created with much
fun, care and love.

Happy art making!

Sannel

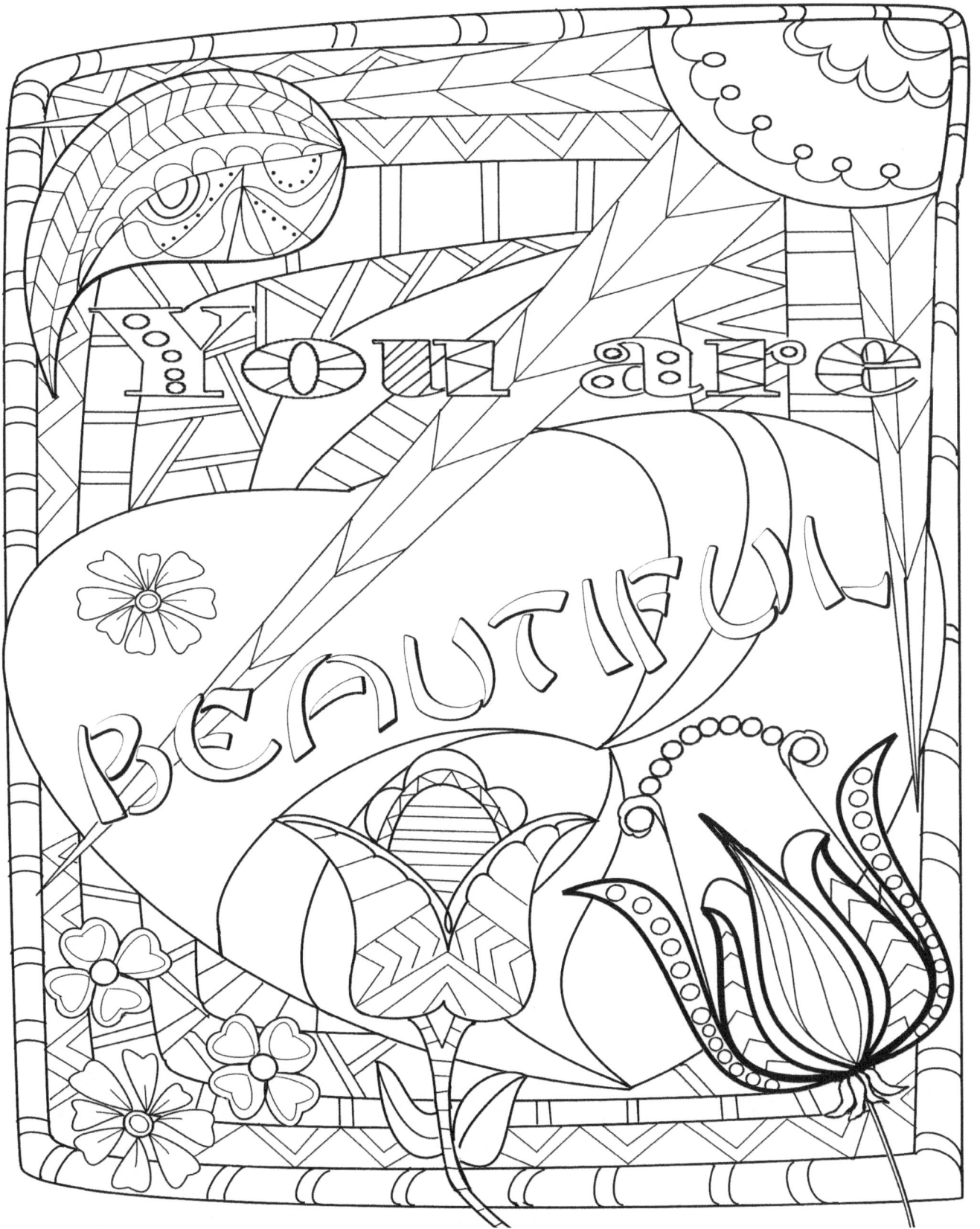

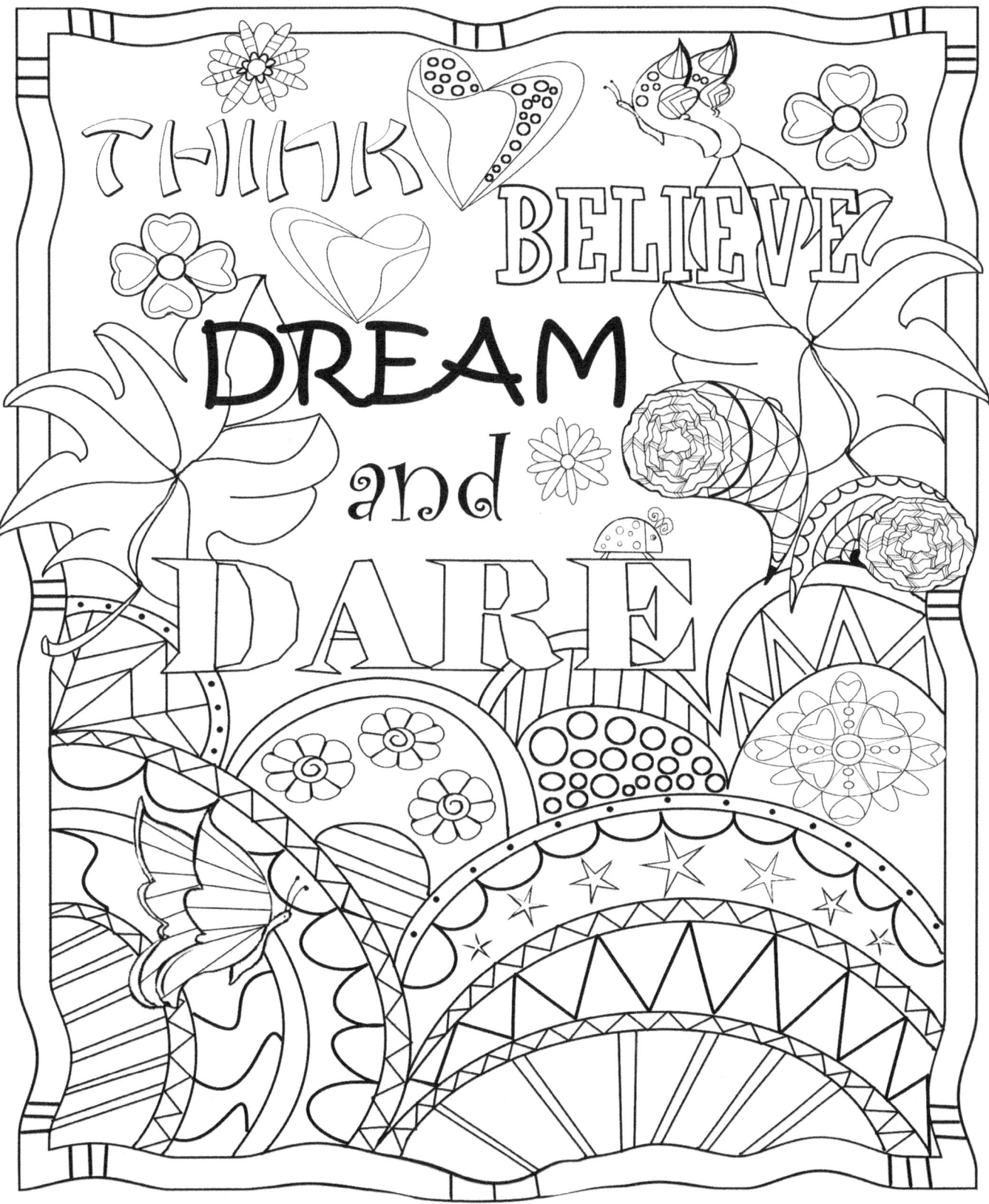

THINK BELIEVE DREAM and DARE

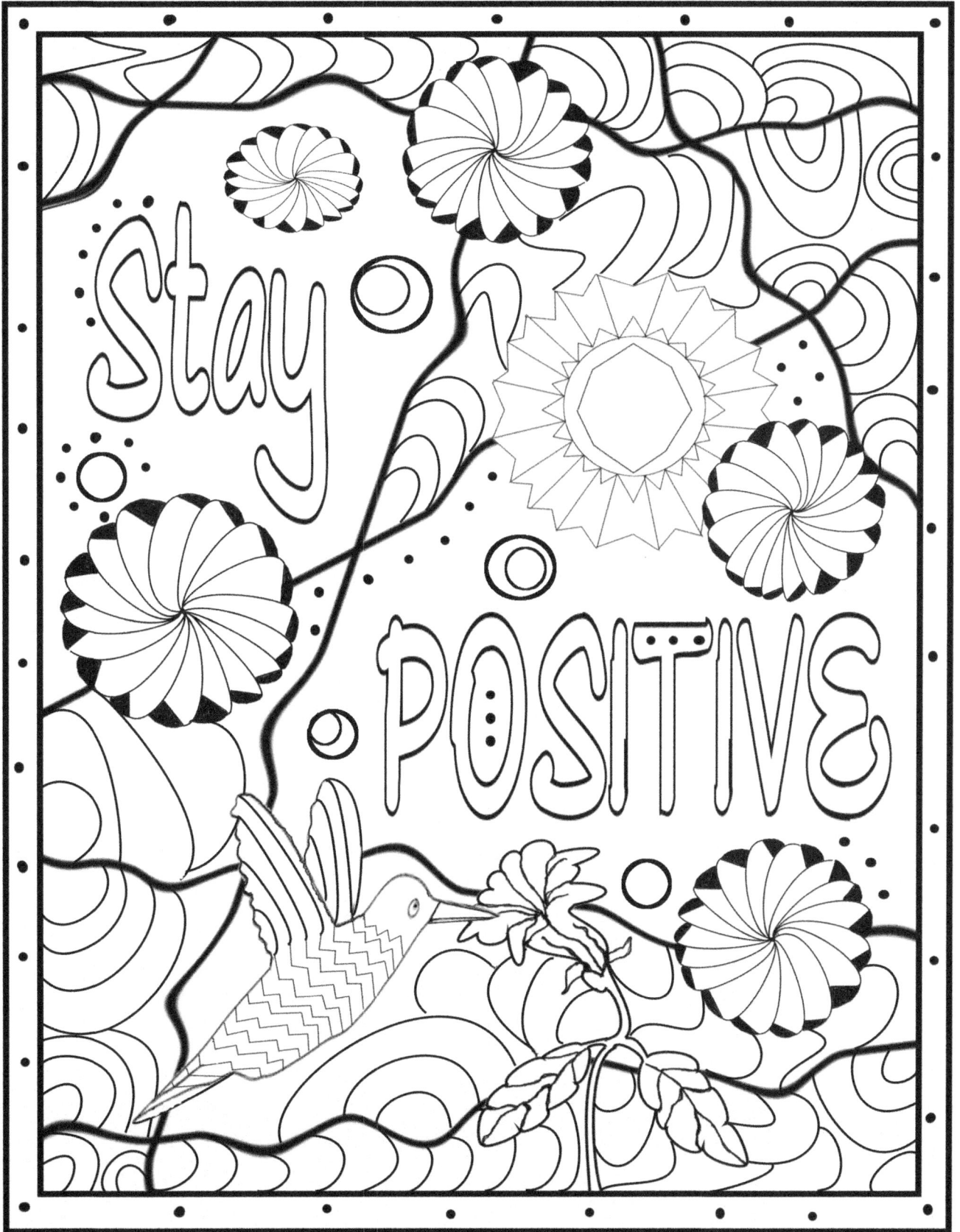

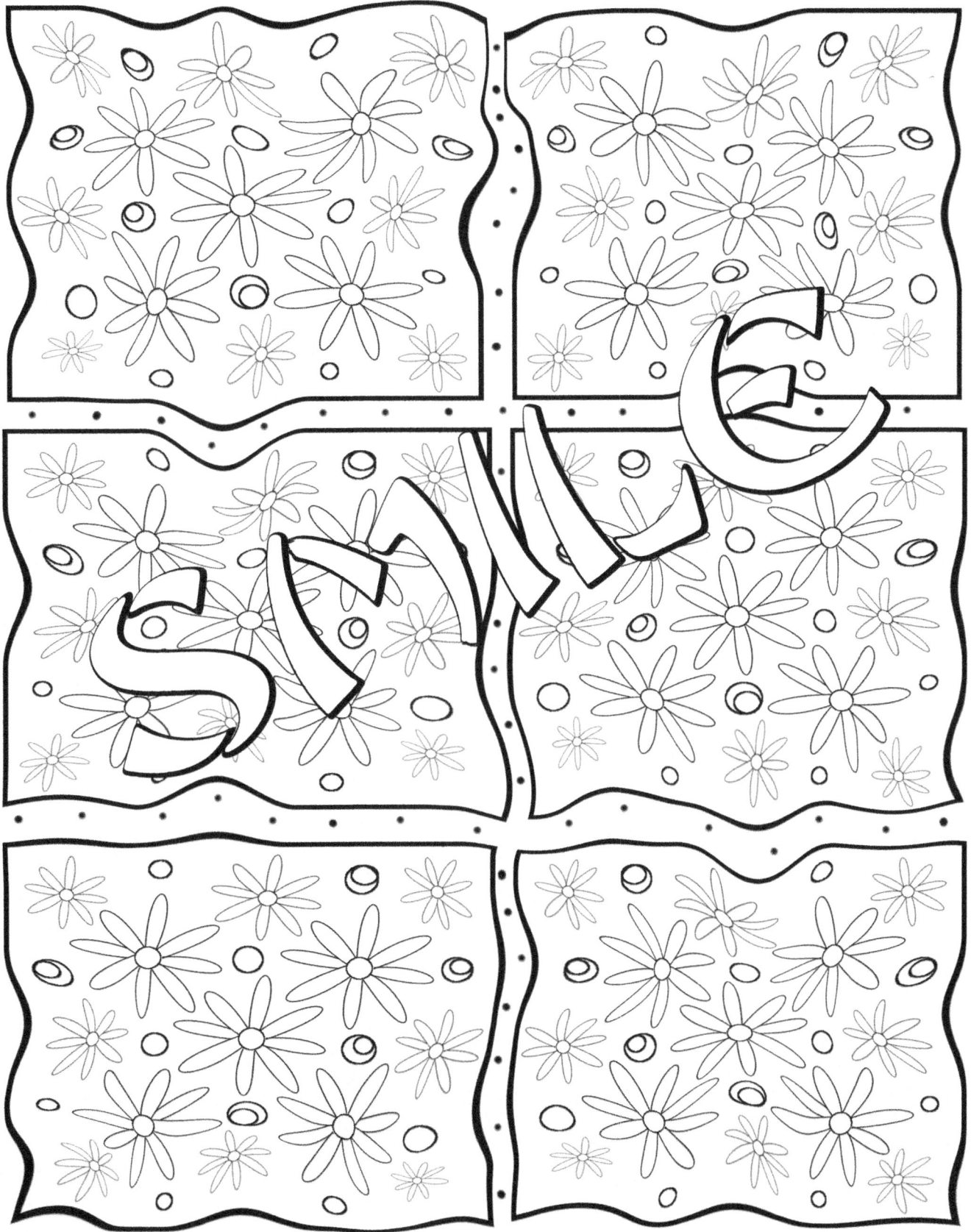

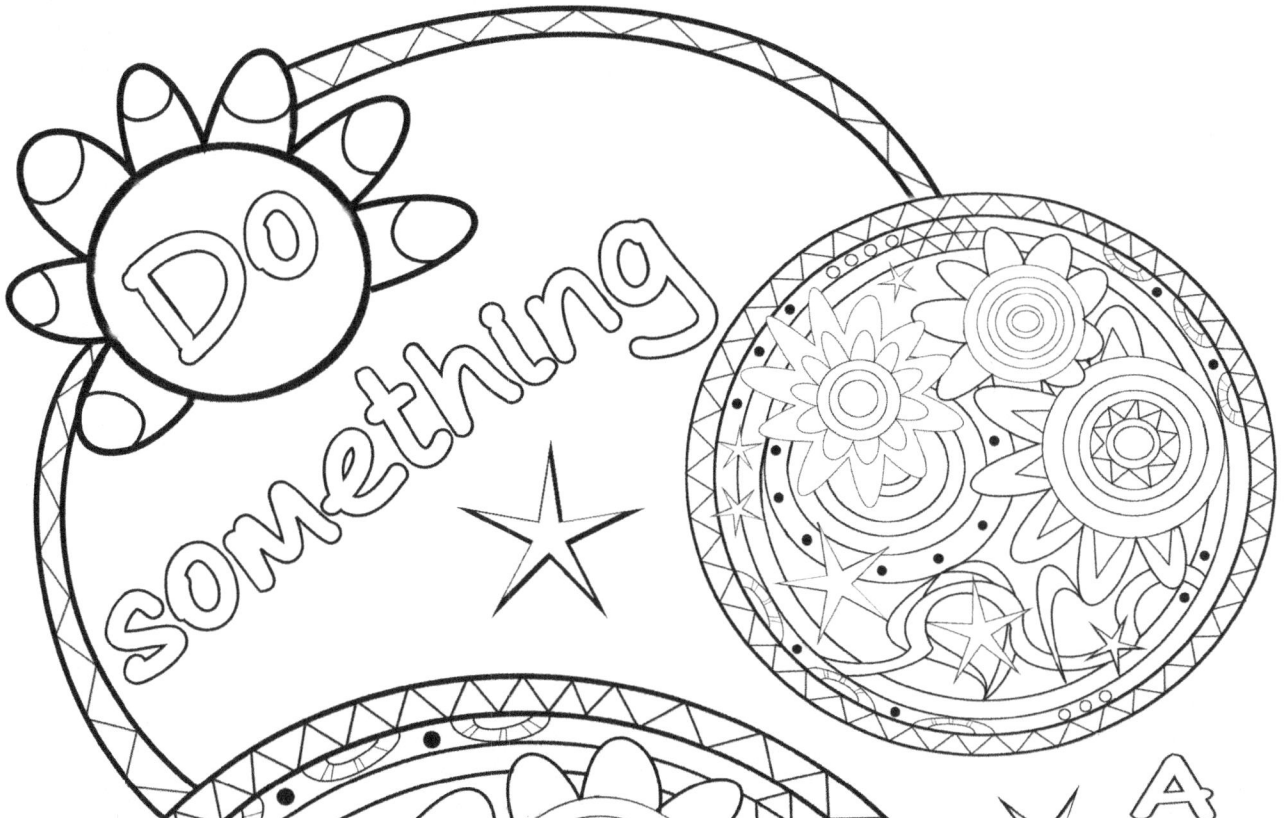

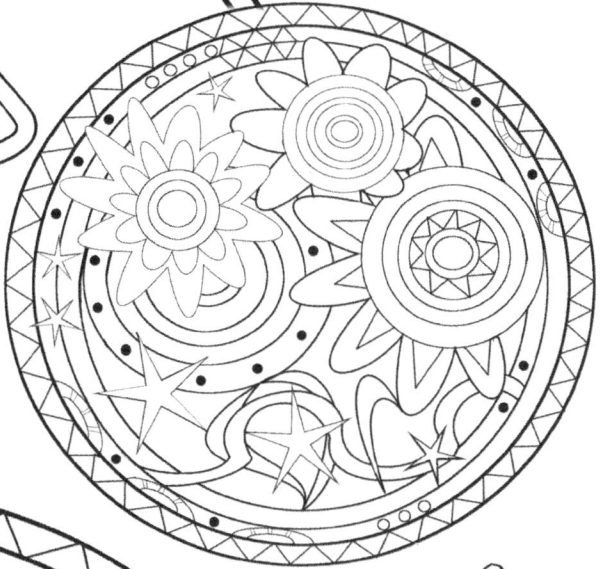

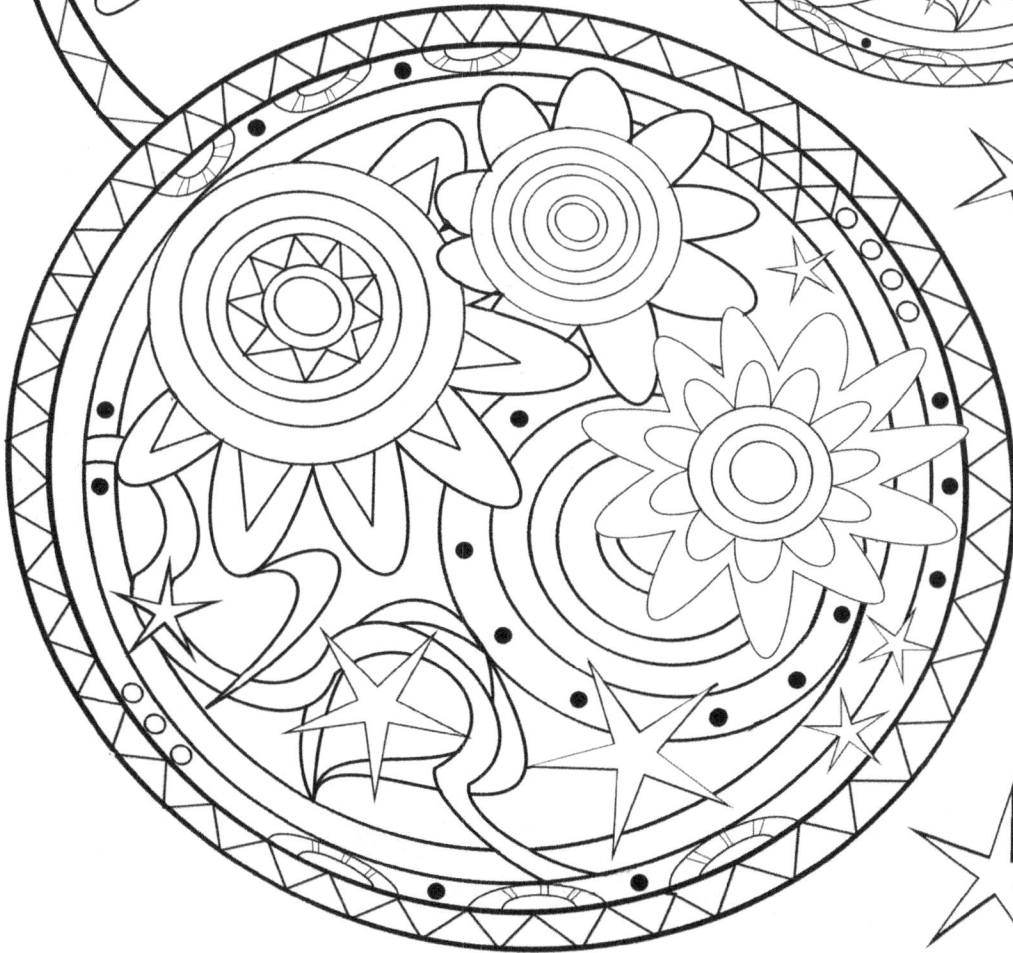

Do something

Amazing

9

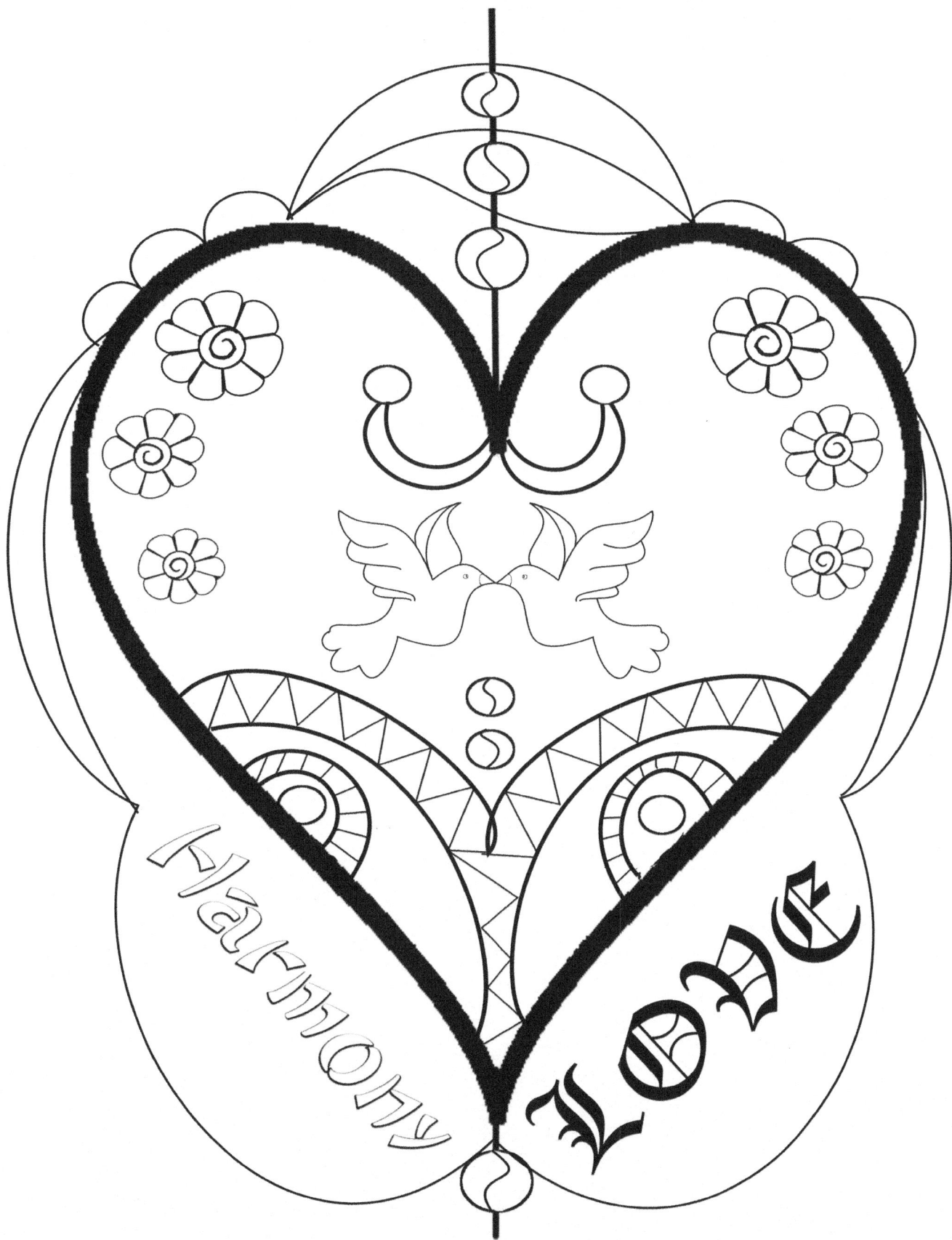

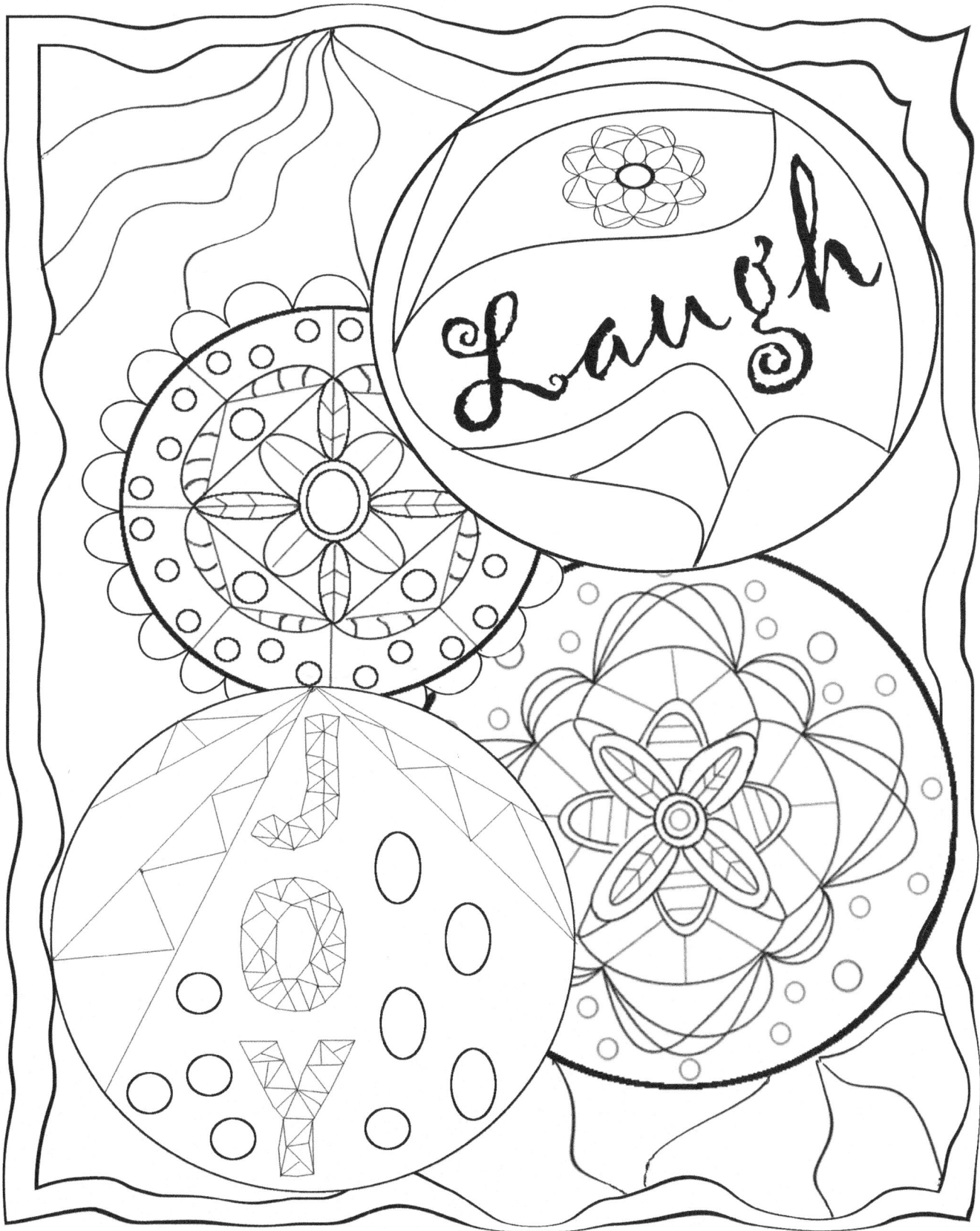

Laugh

JOY

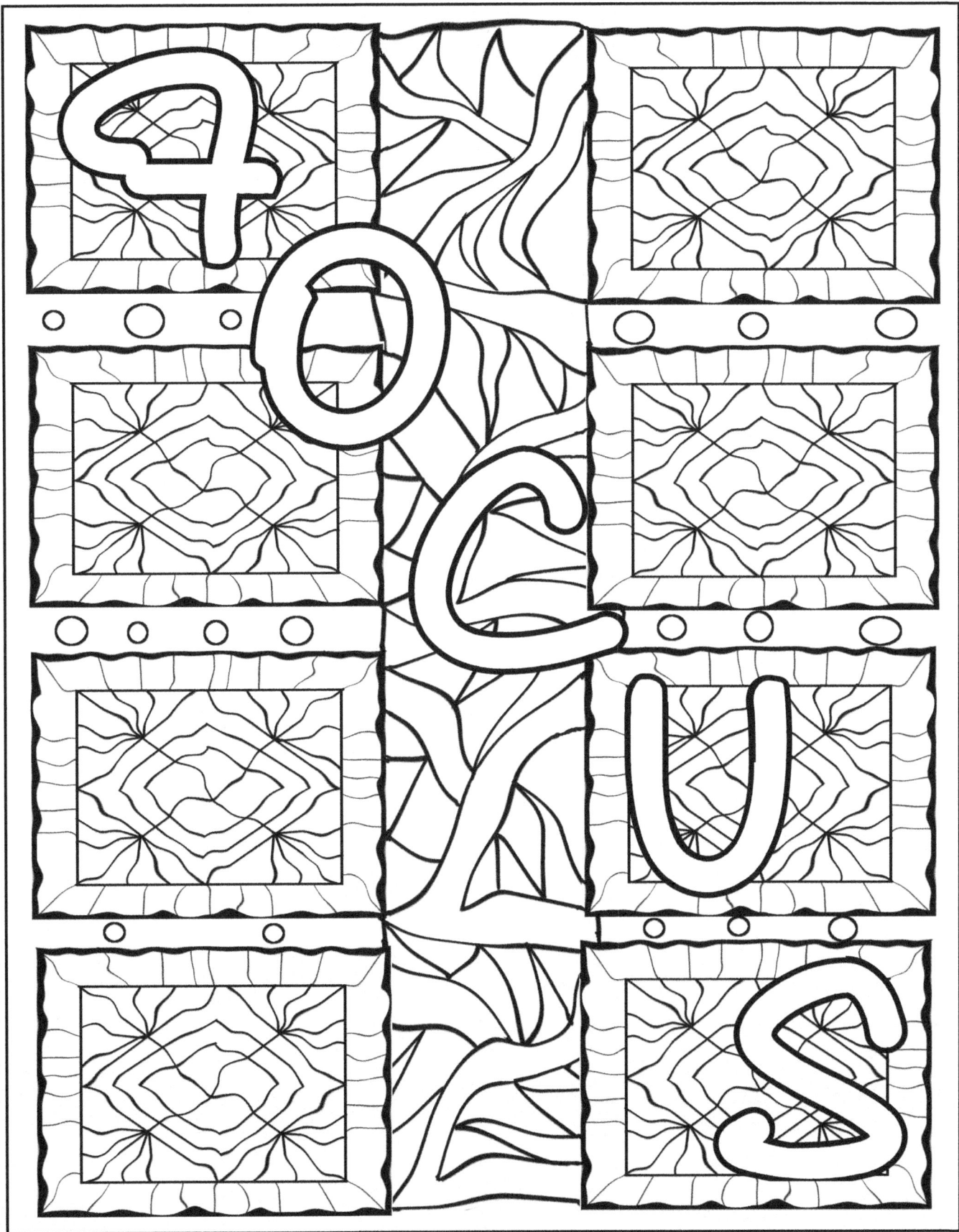

FOCUS

LIVE LIFE with arms WIDE OPEN

Only in the darkness can you see the STARS

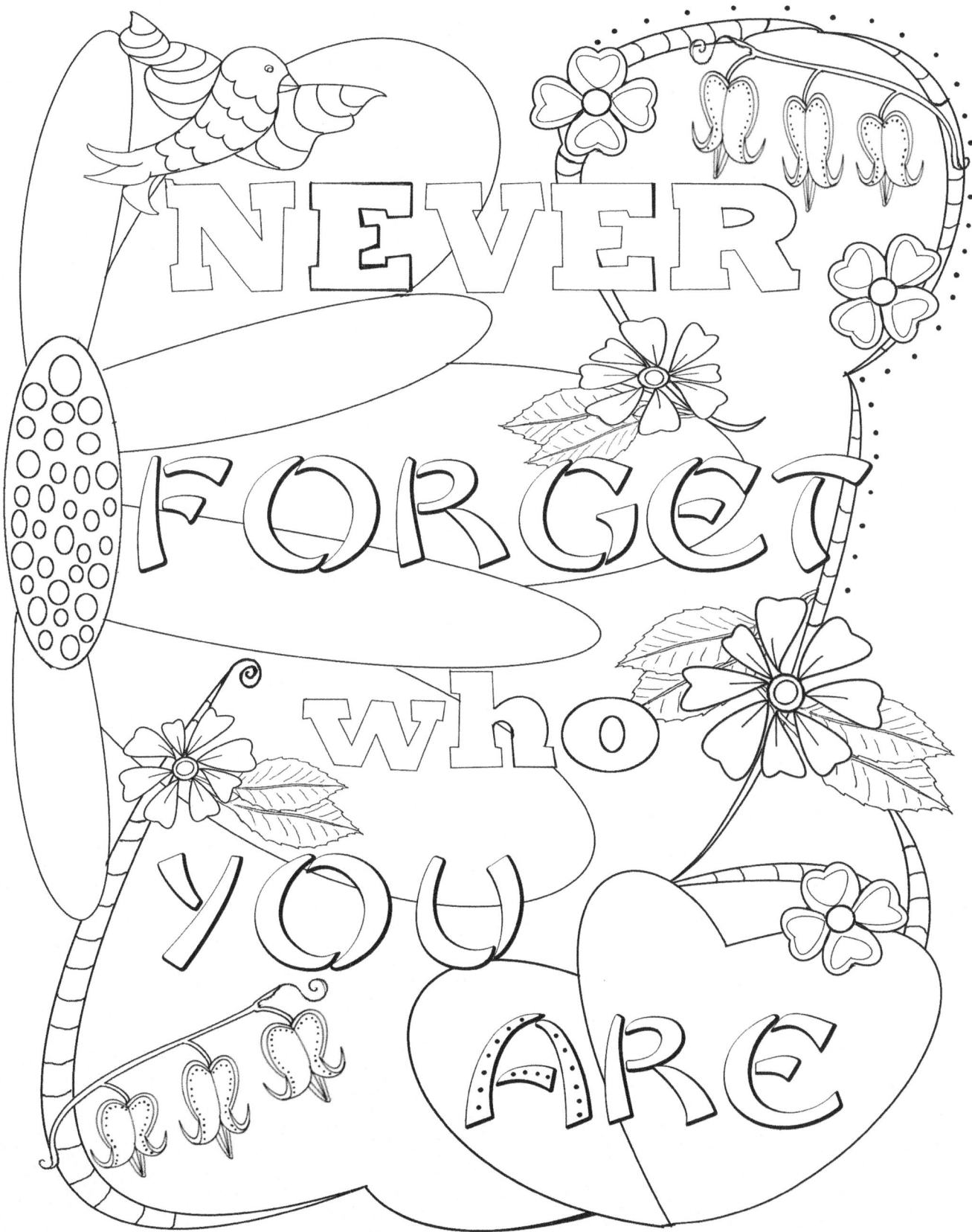

NEVER FORGET who YOU ARE

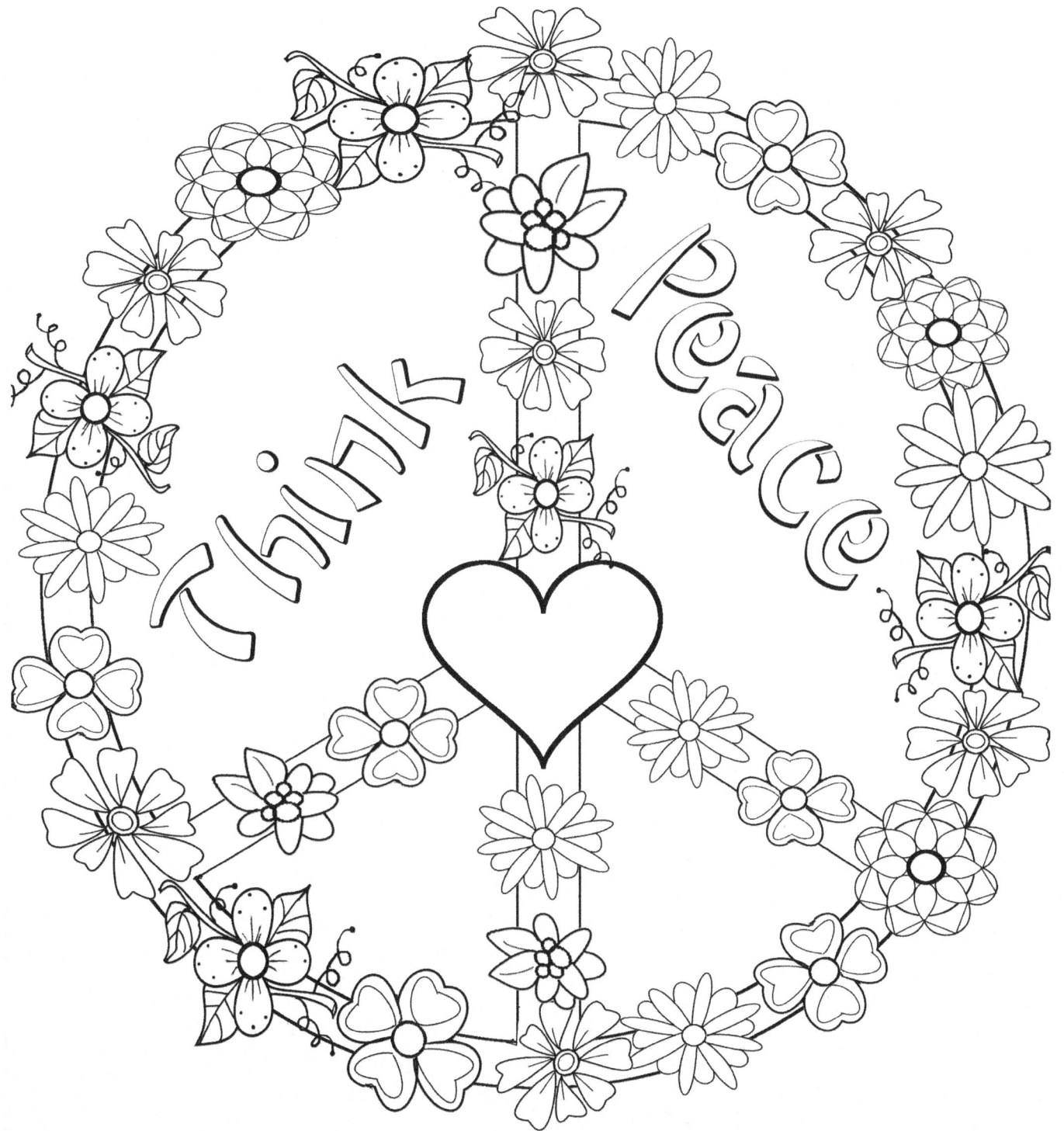

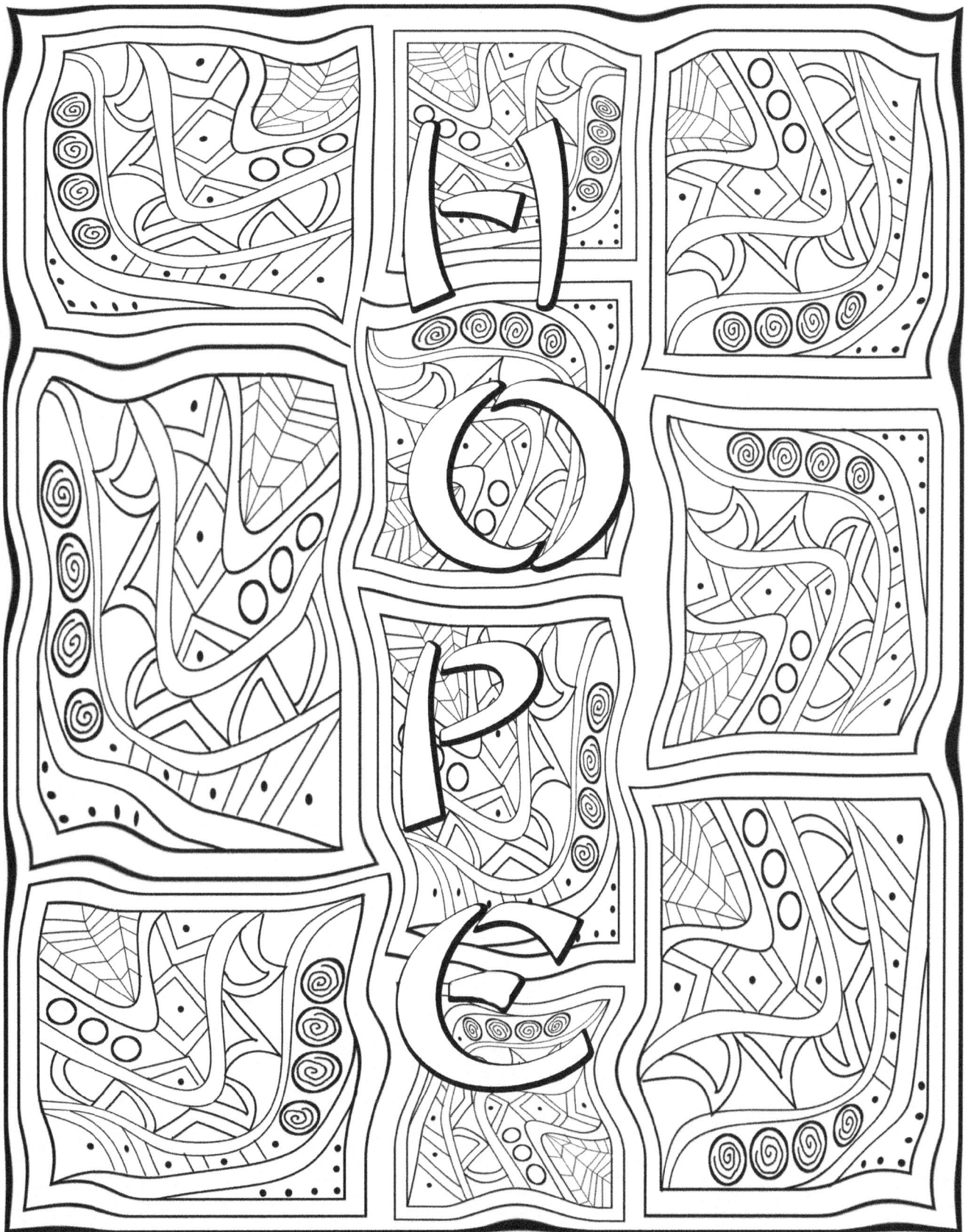

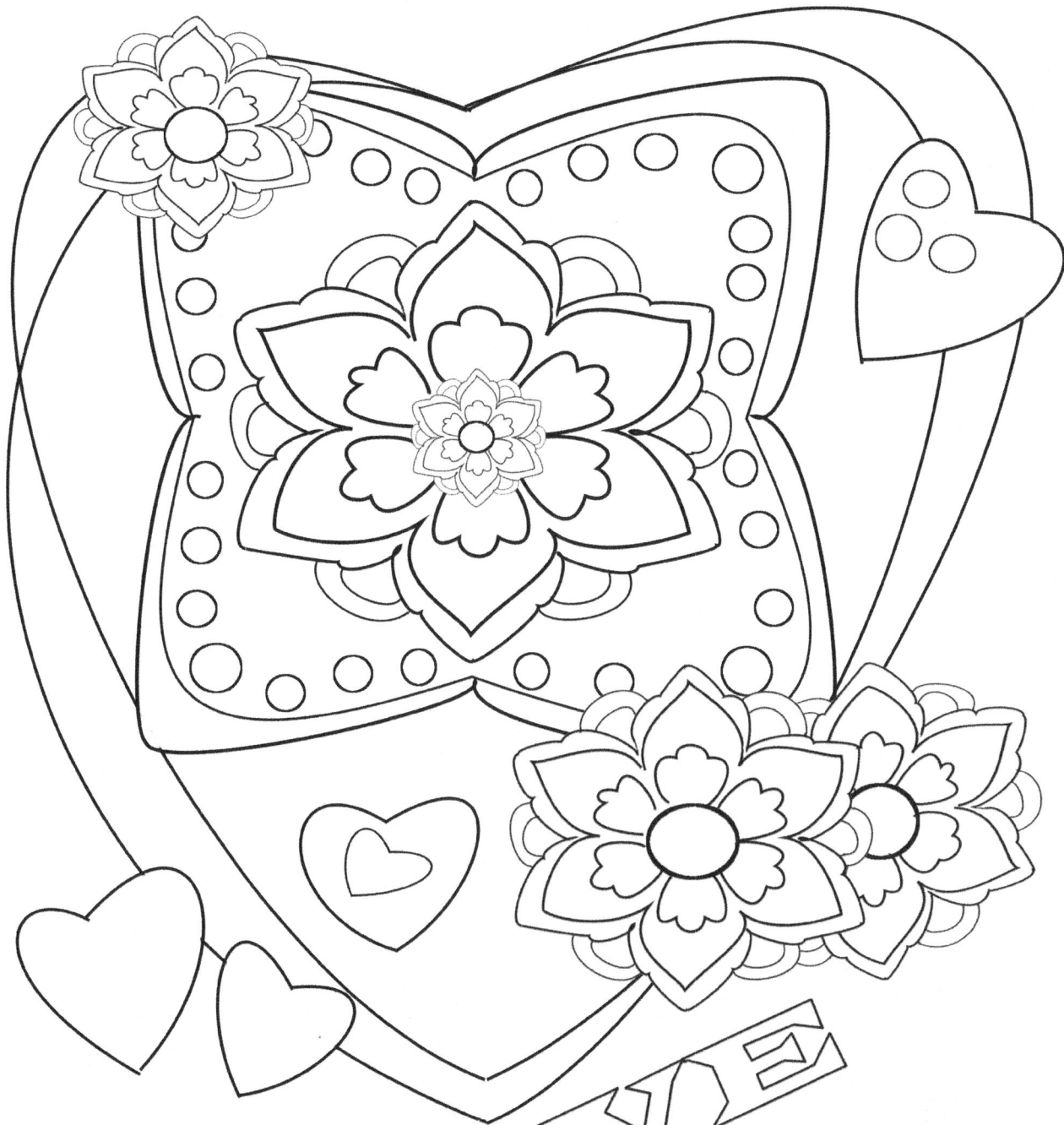

LIVE love LAUGH

TODAY IS THE PERFECT *day* to be HAPPY

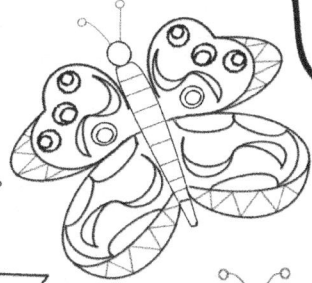
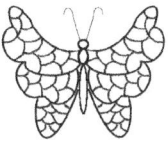
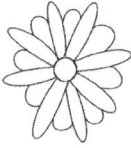
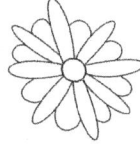
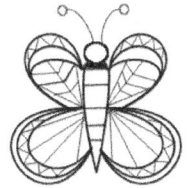
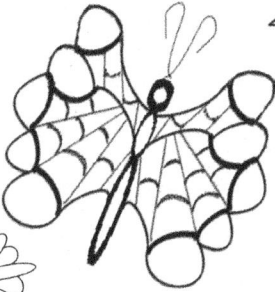
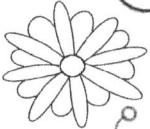
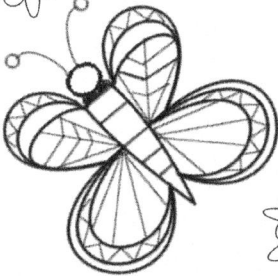
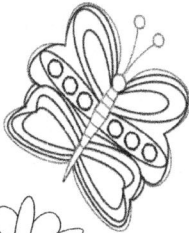
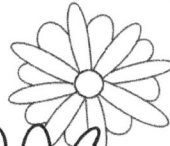
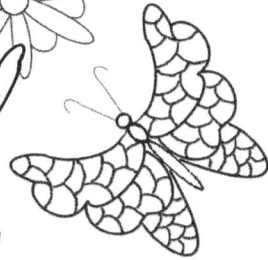
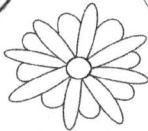
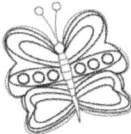
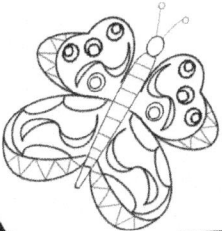
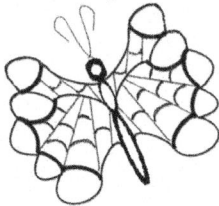
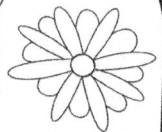

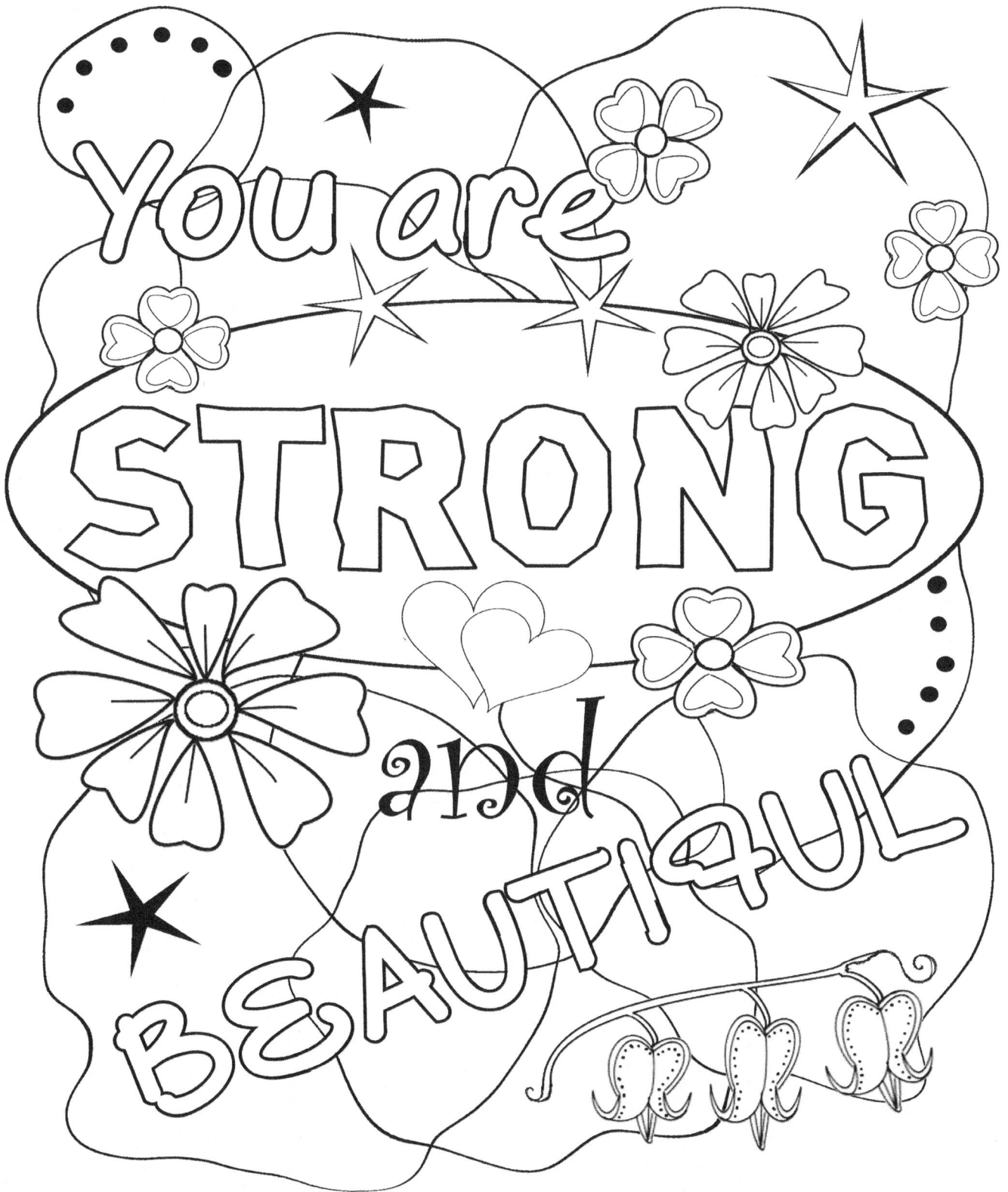

You are STRONG and BEAUTIQUL

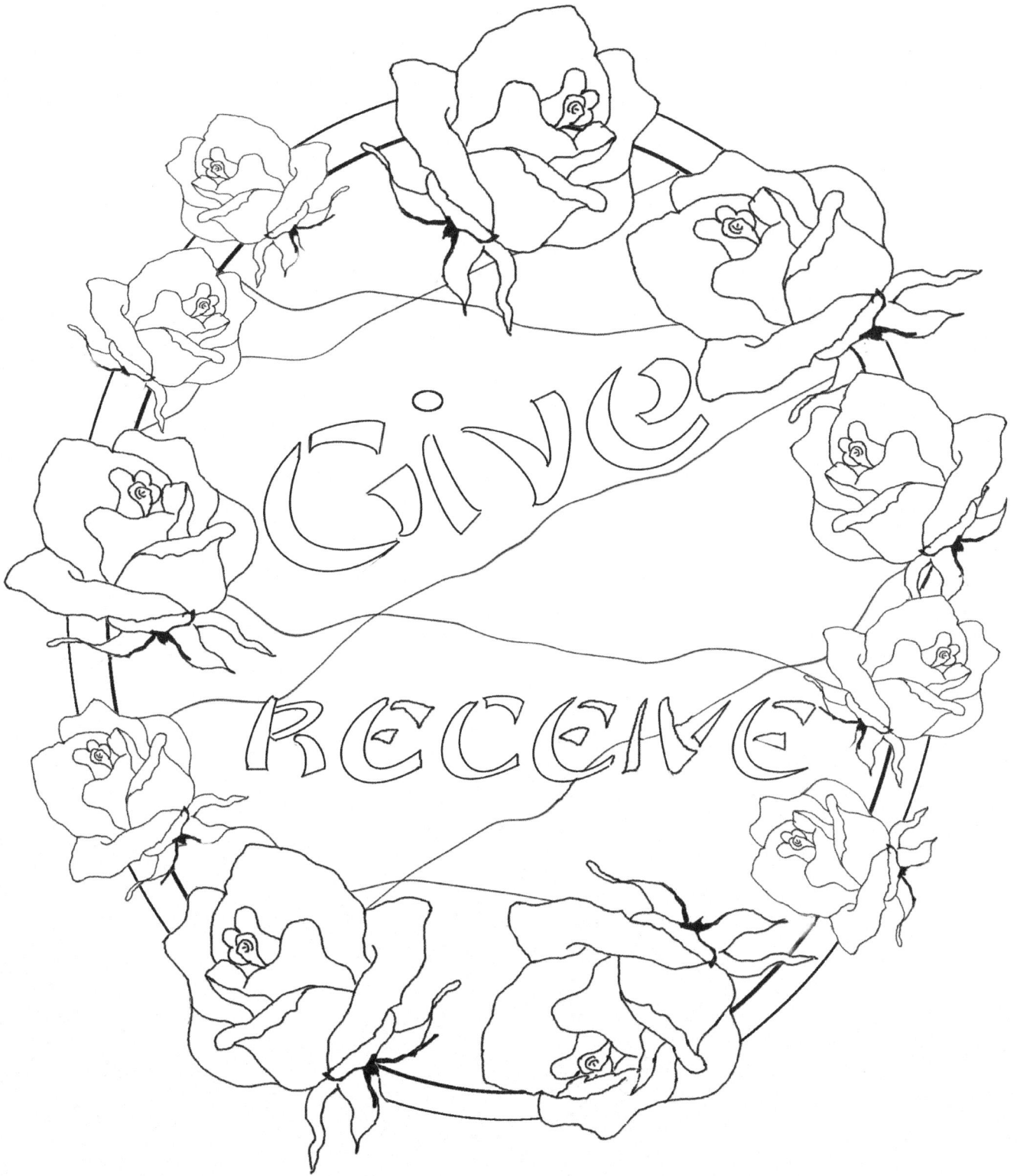

Give

RECEIVE

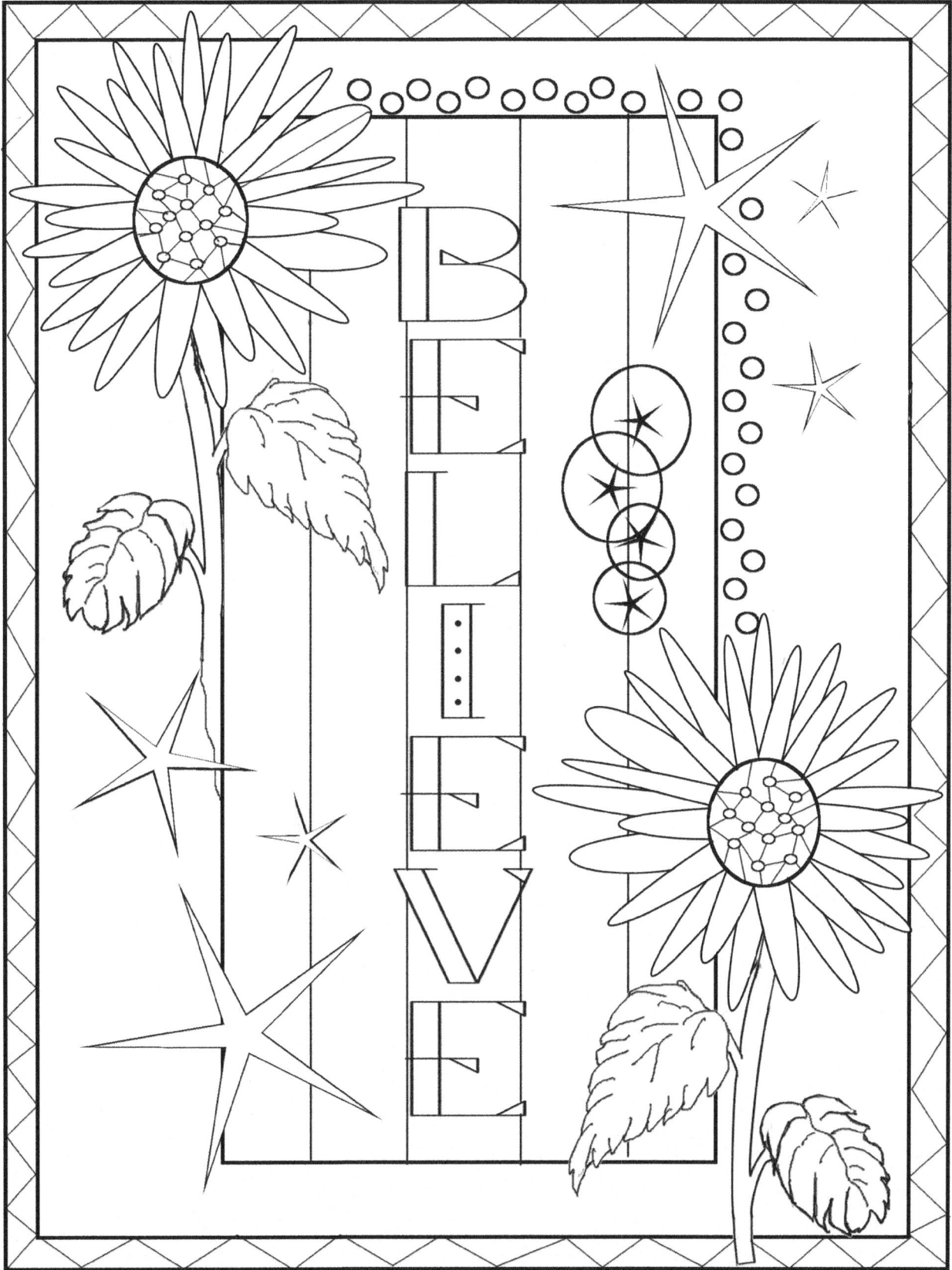

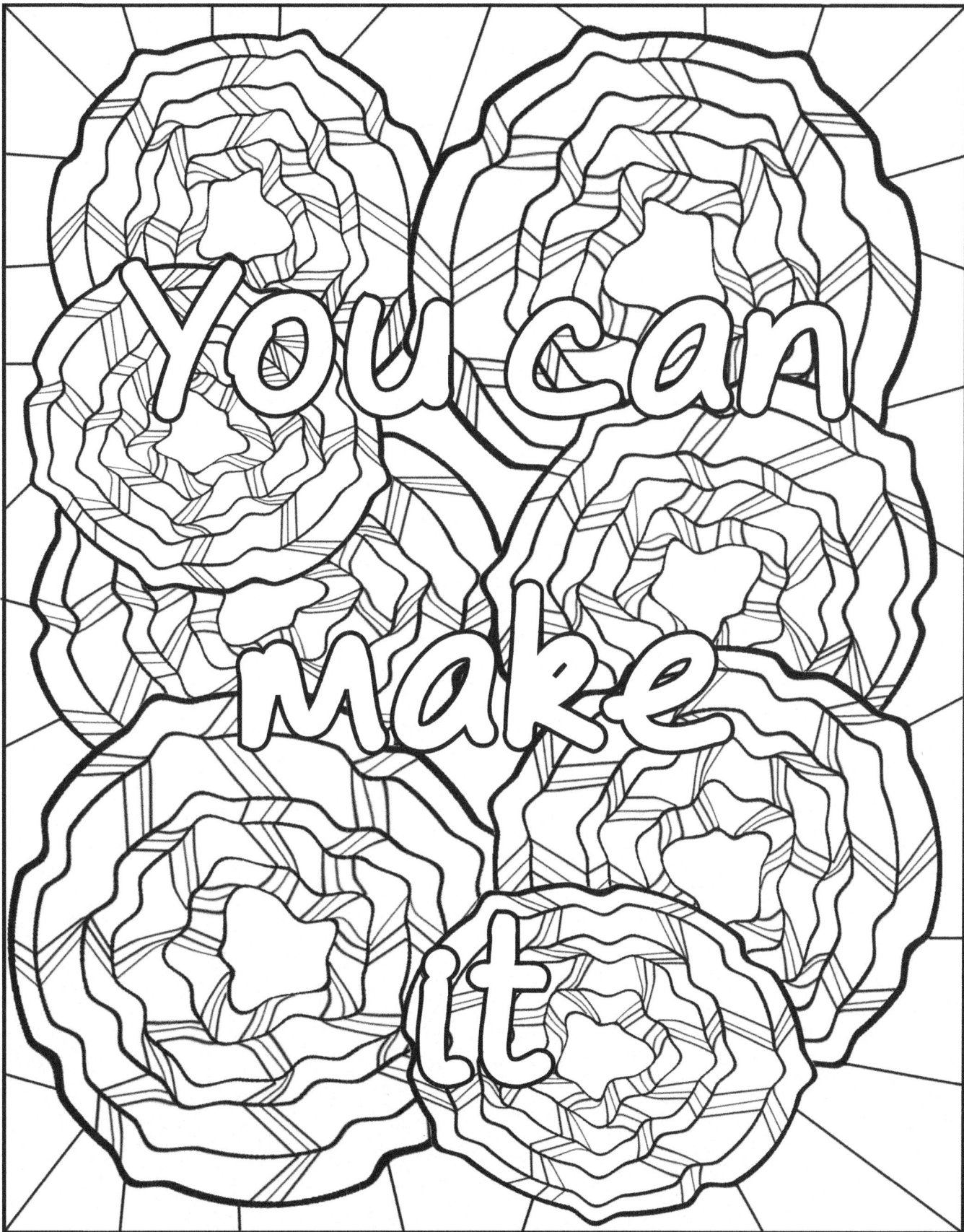

You can make it

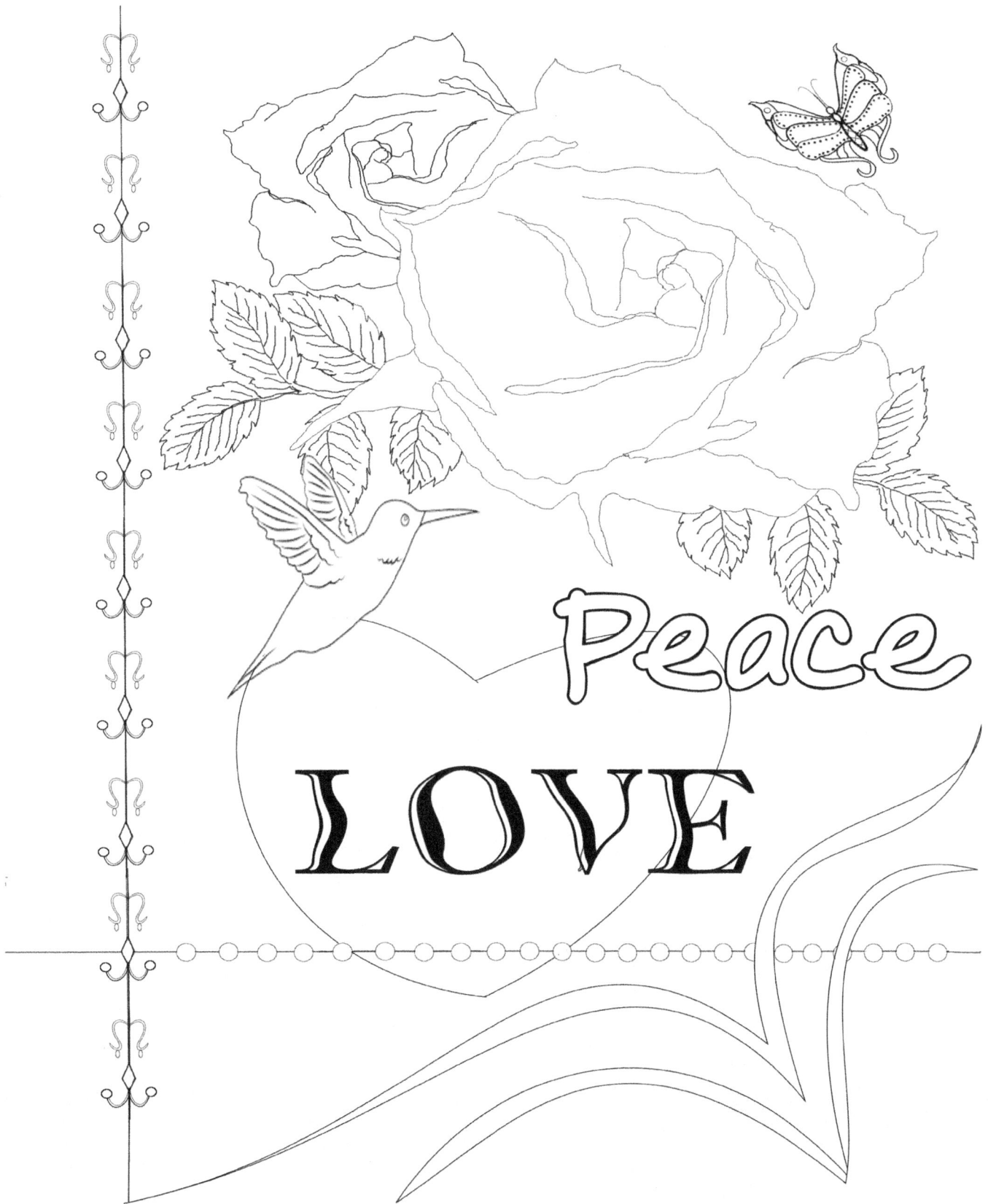

Peace

LOVE

39

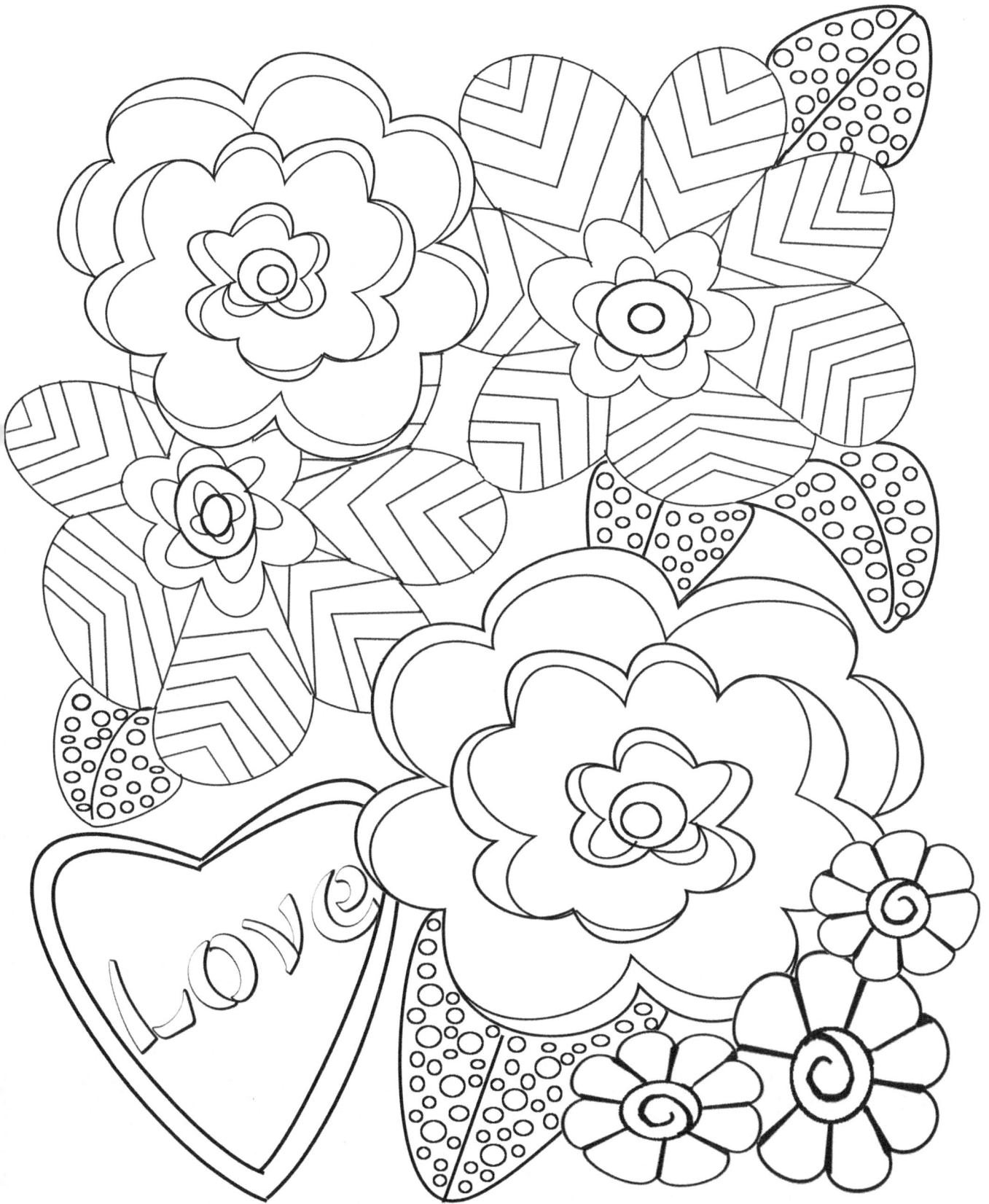

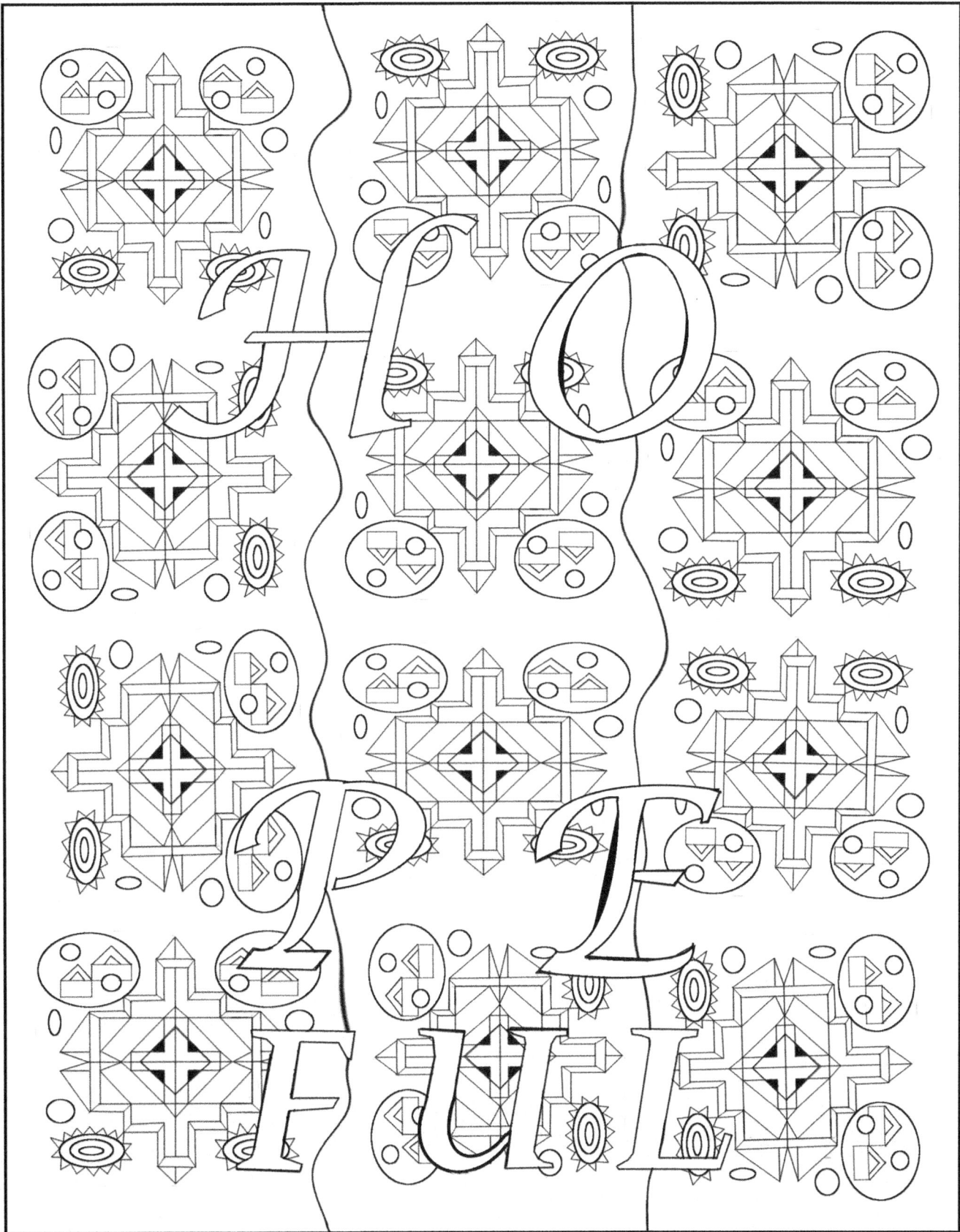

HOPEFUL

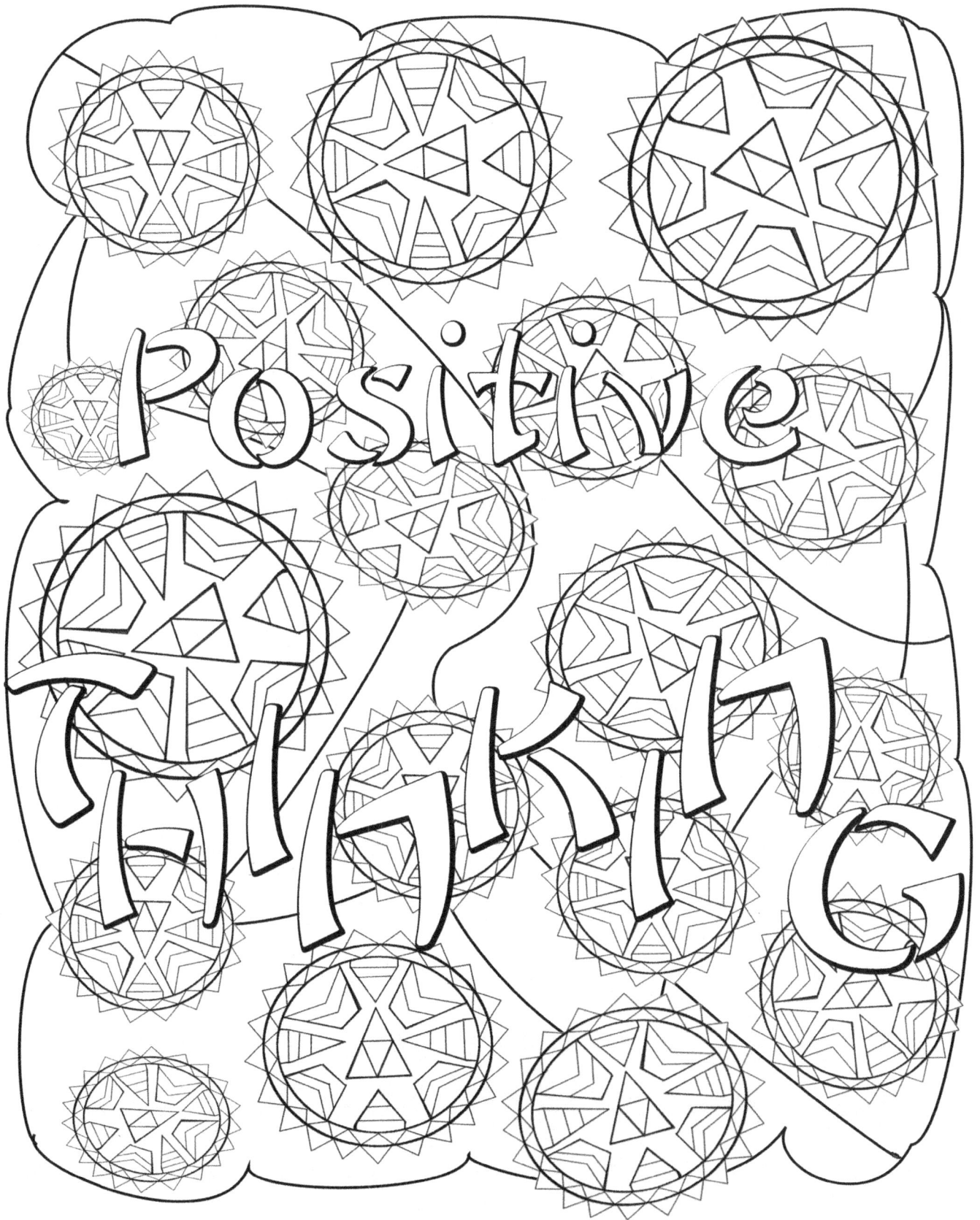

Positive Thinking

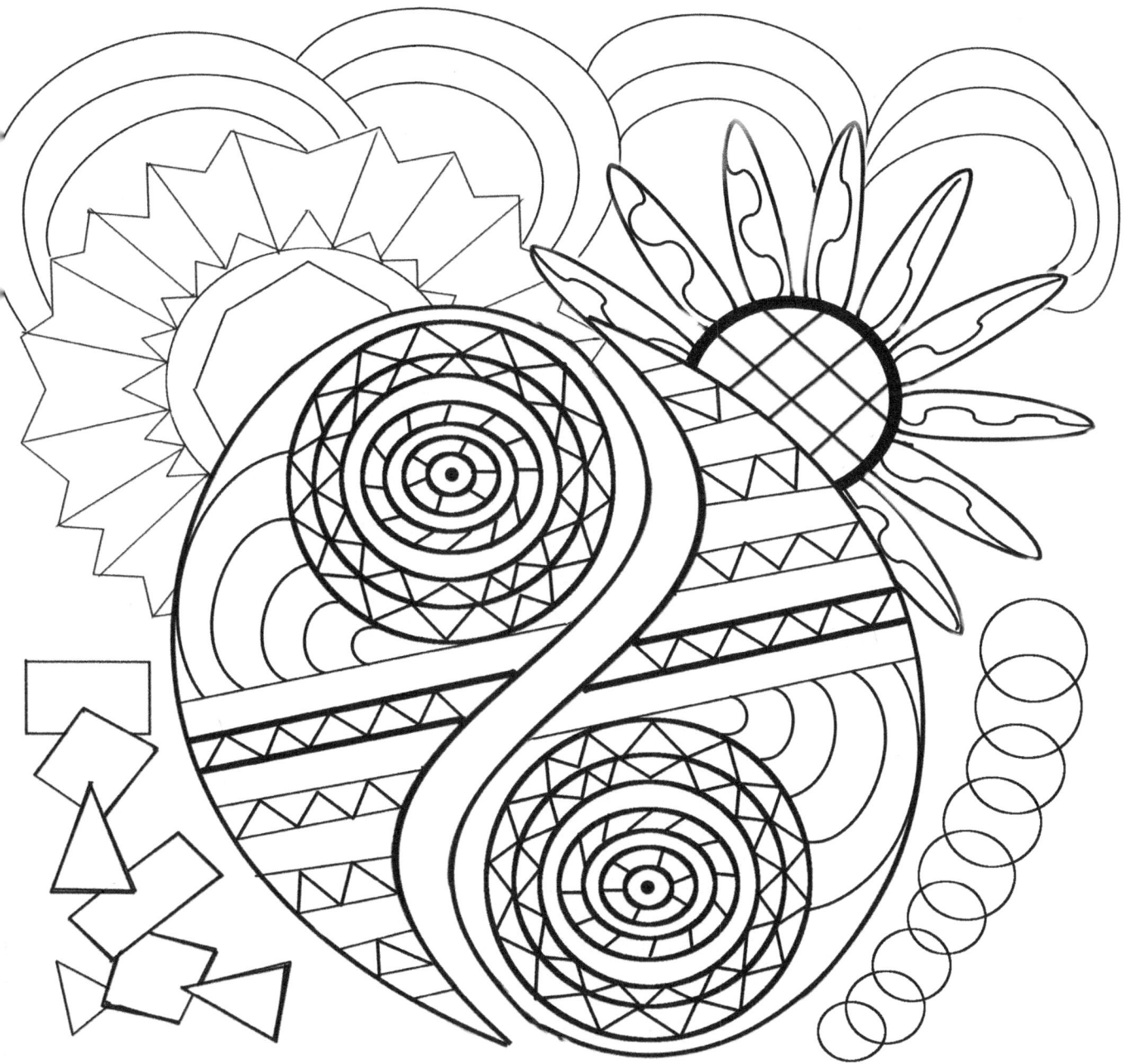

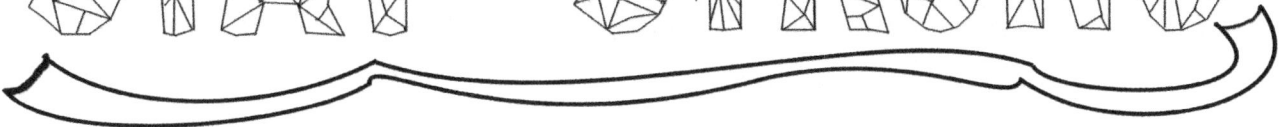

STAY STRONG

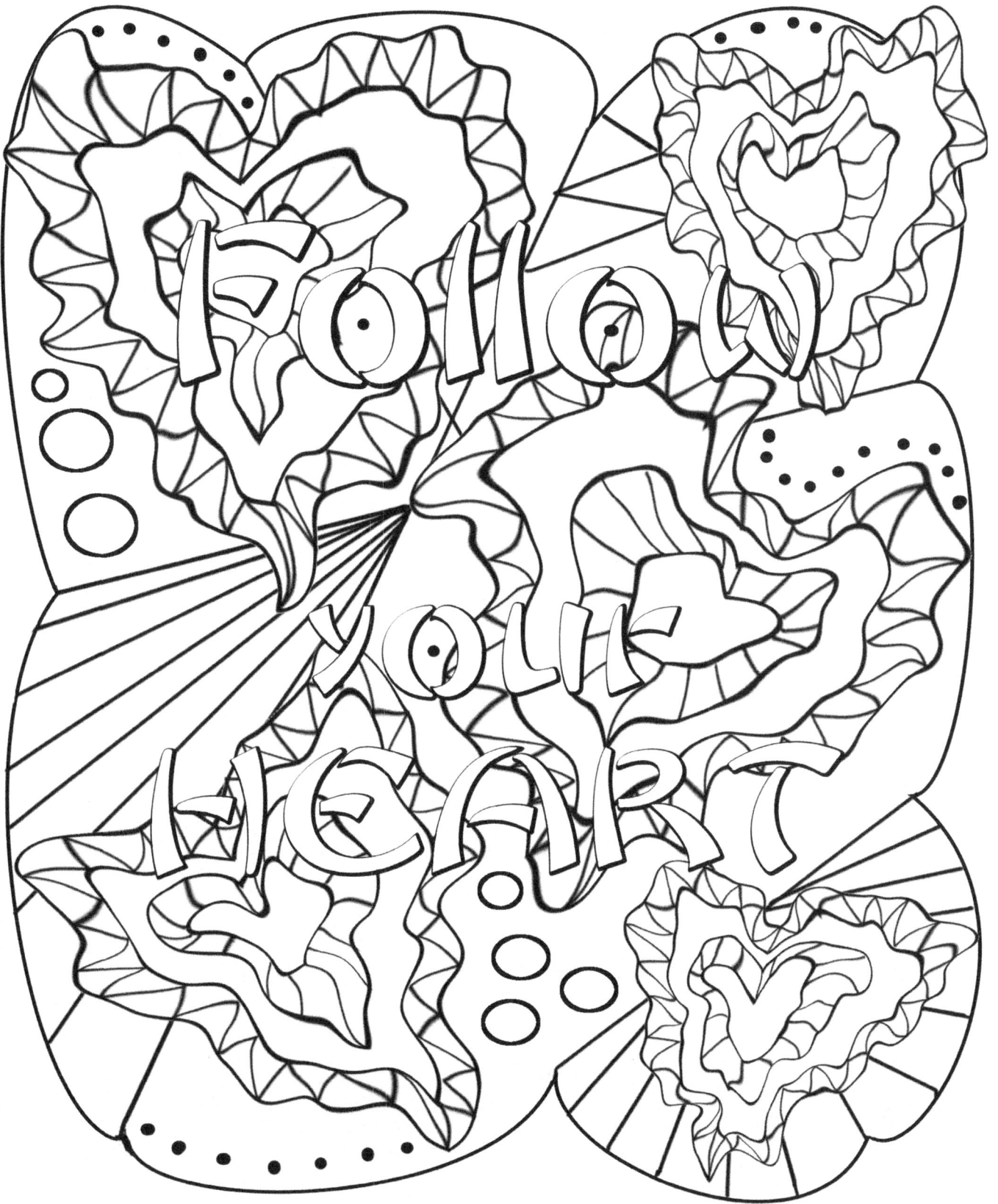

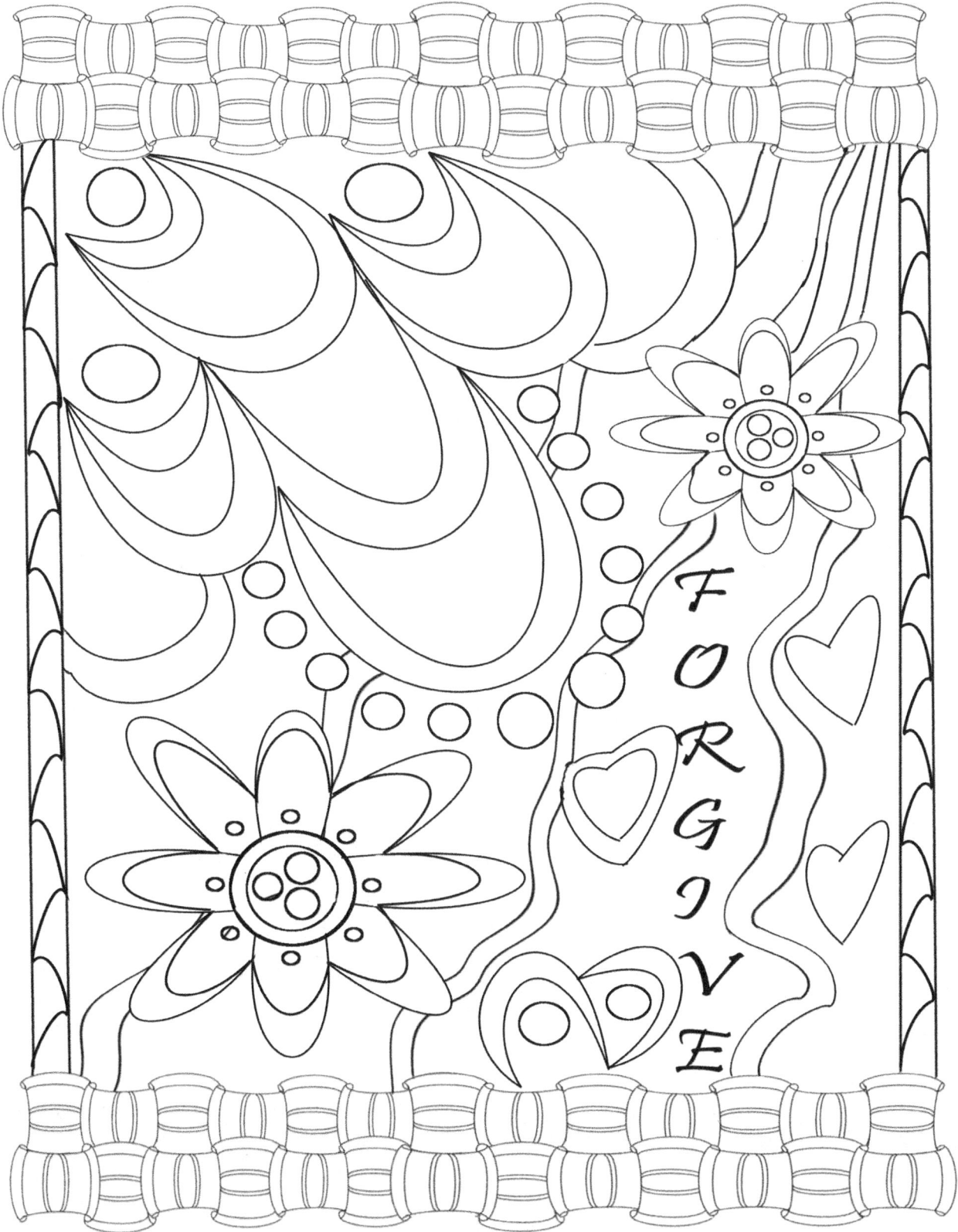

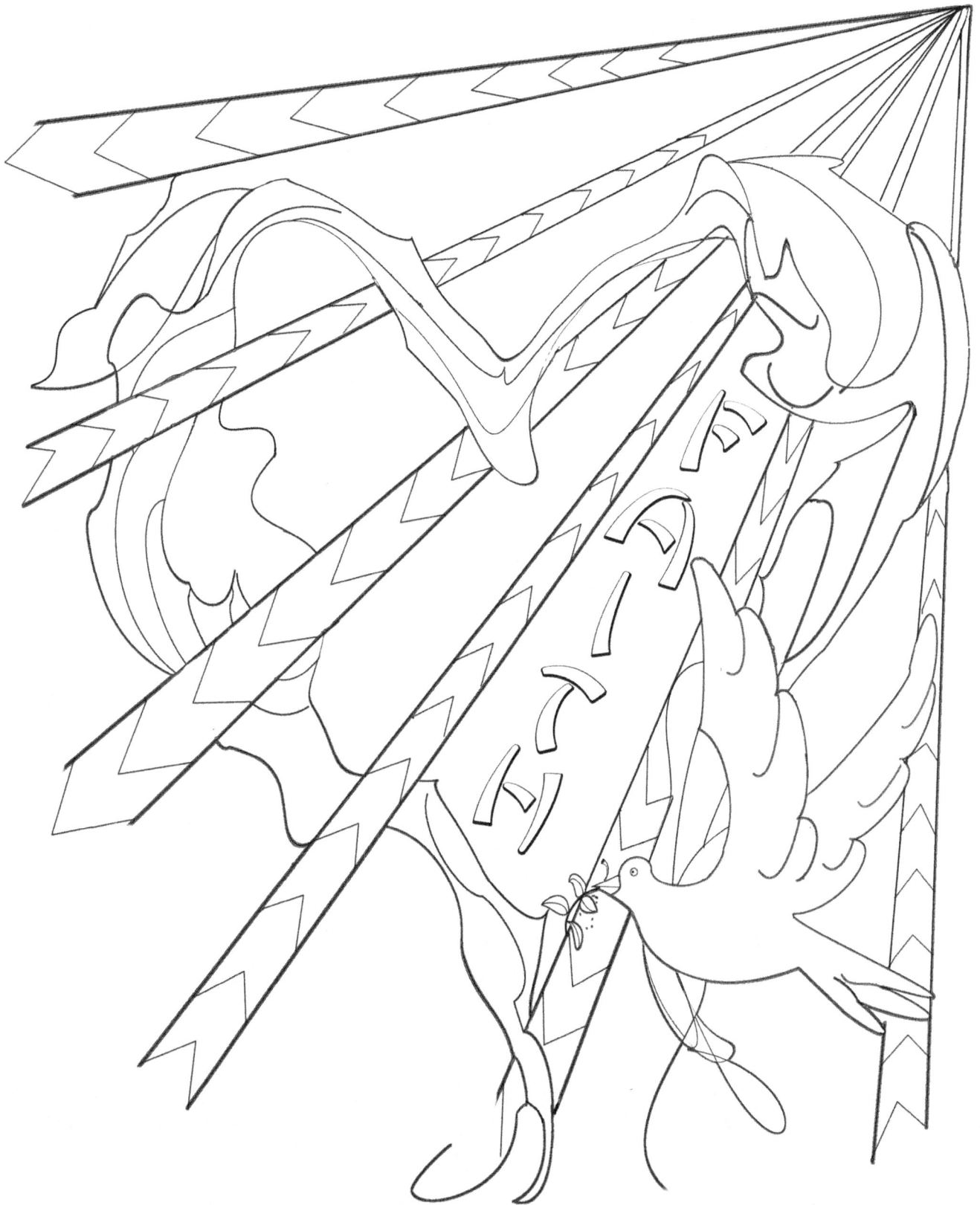

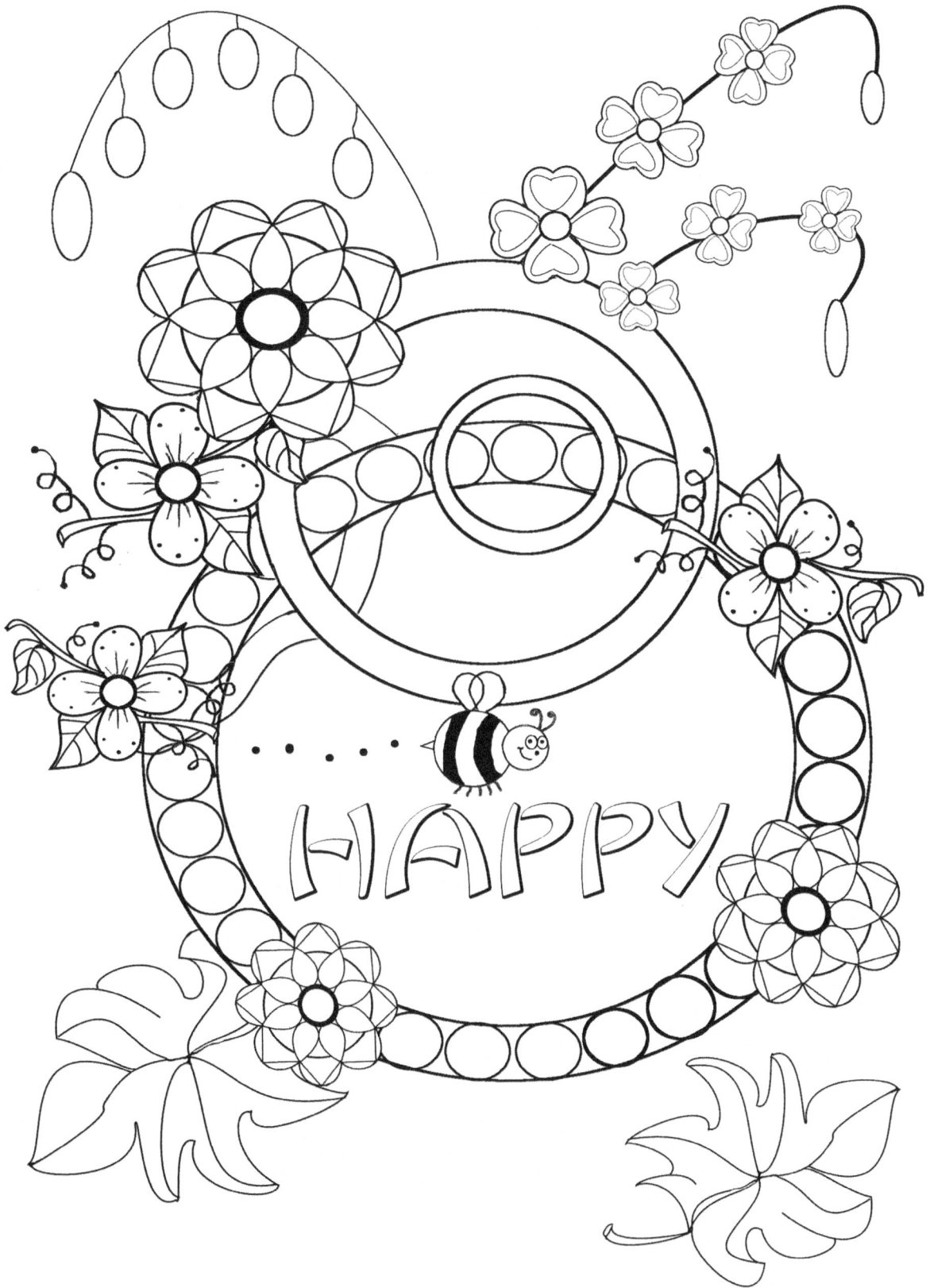

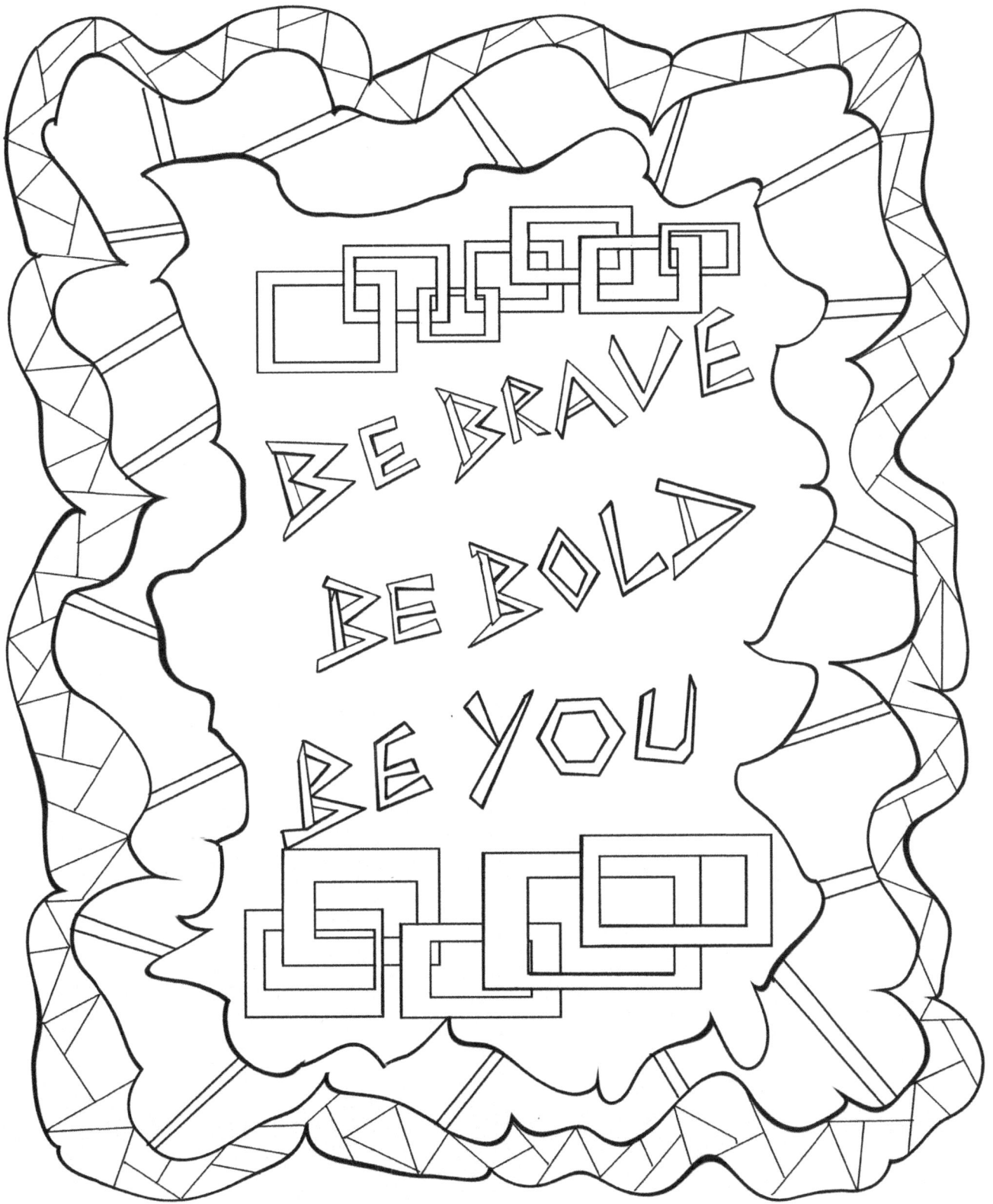

BE BRAVE
BE BOLD
BE YOU

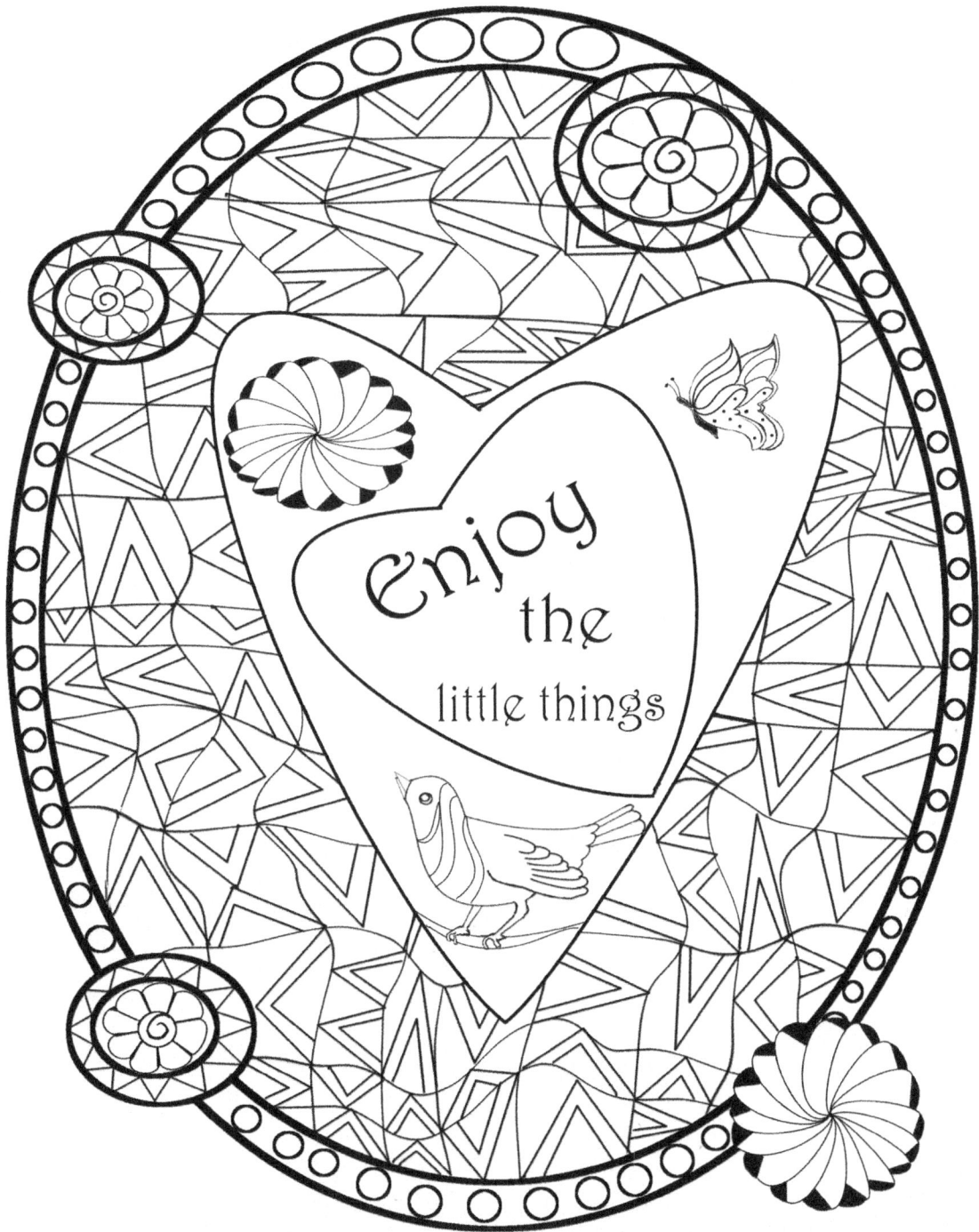

Enjoy the little things

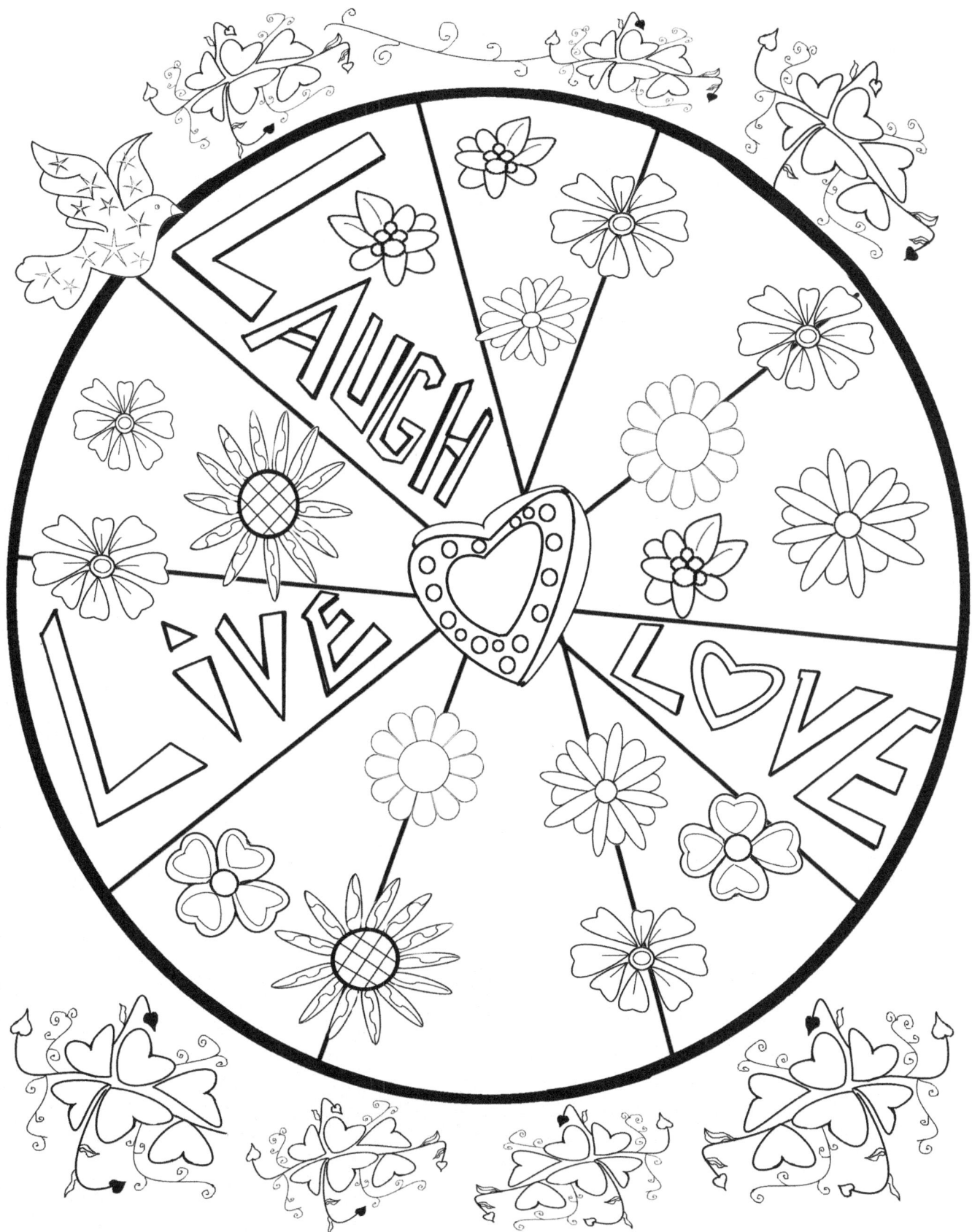

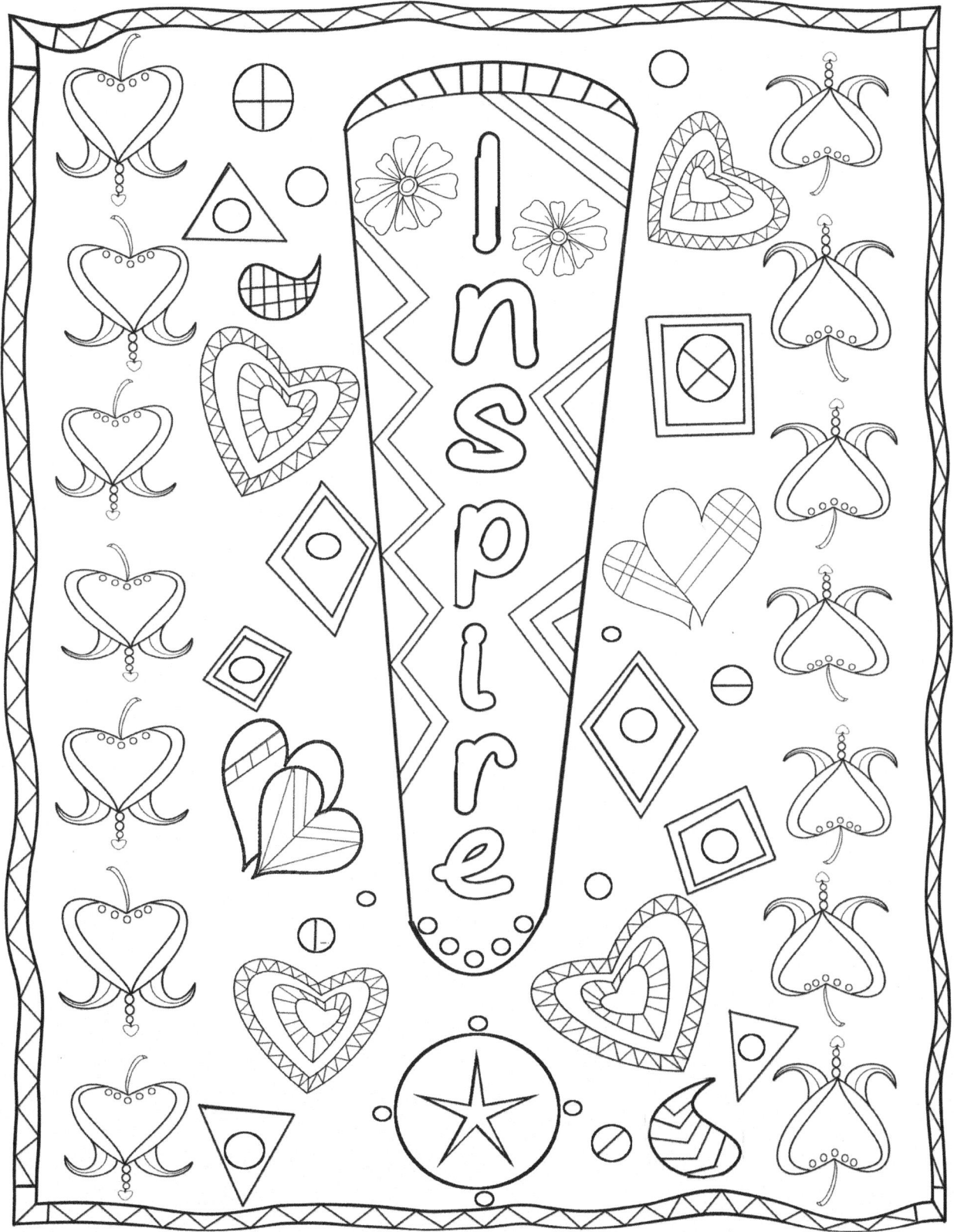

Inspire

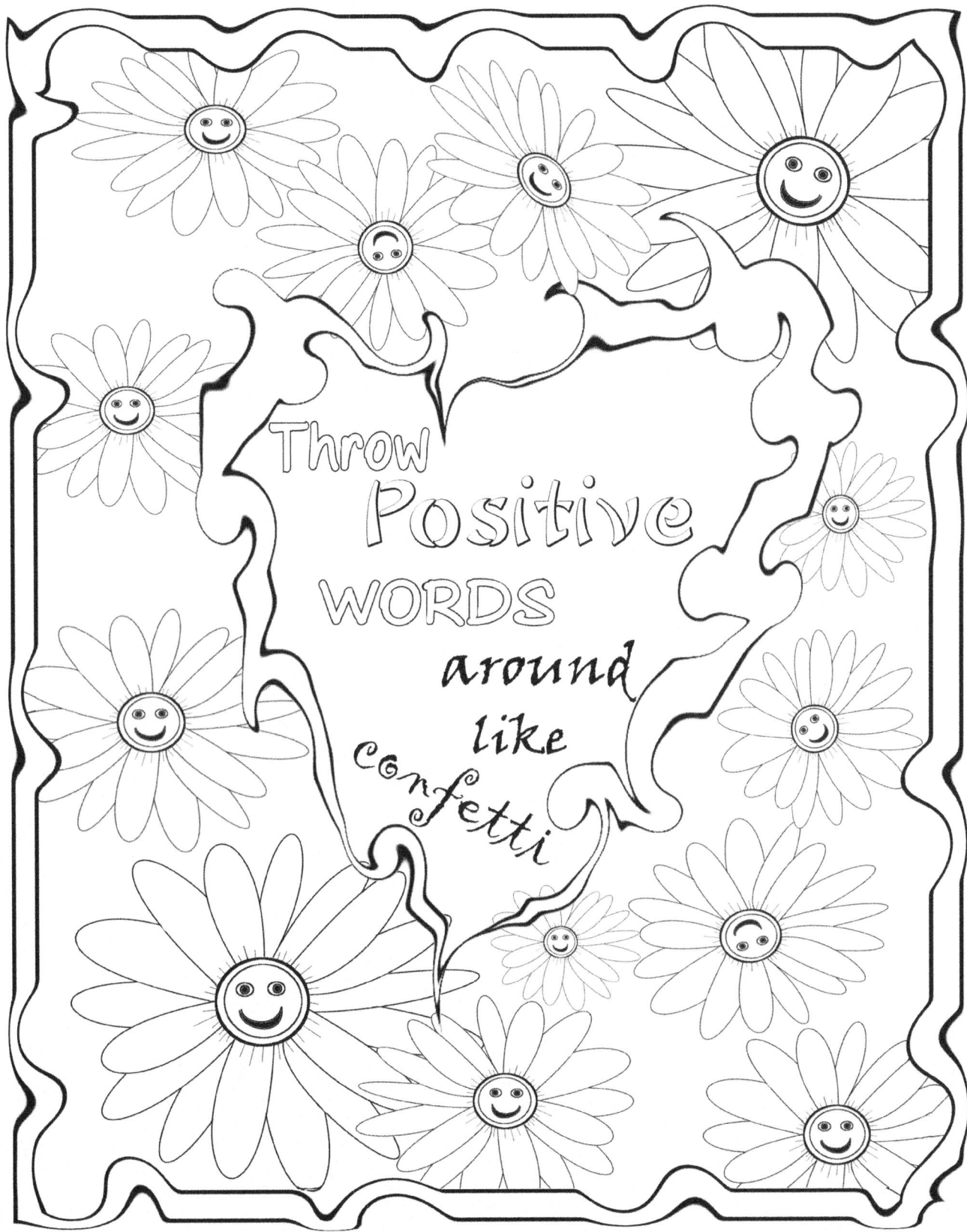

Throw Positive WORDS around like confetti

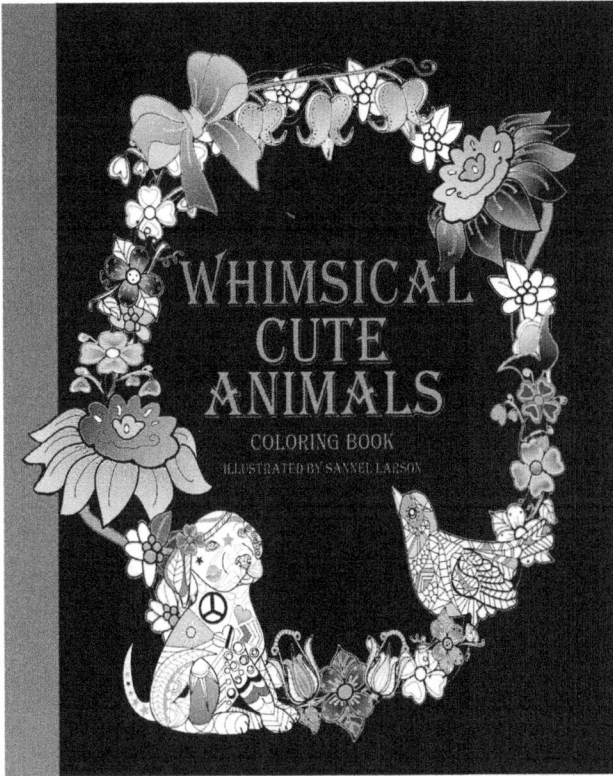

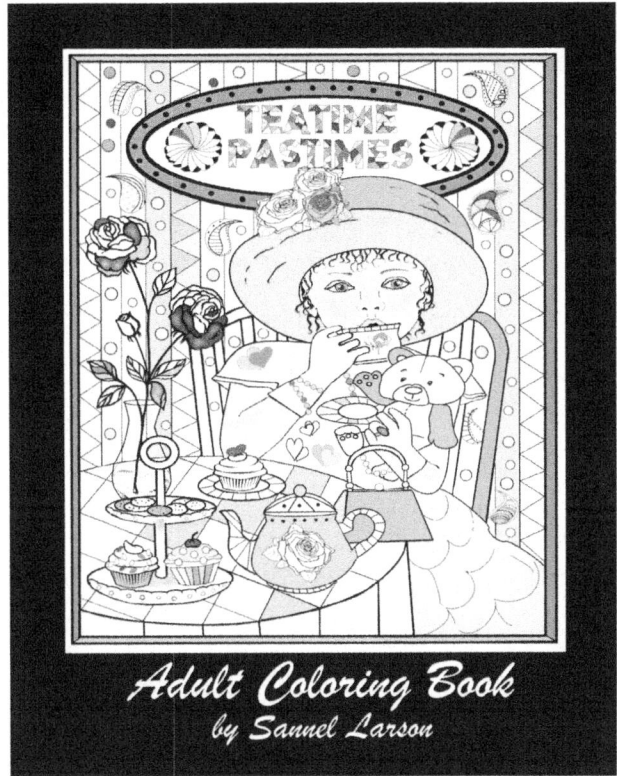

Here are a few more coloring books by
Sannel Larson, featuring beautiful,
imaginative illustrations to color. They can
be found on amazon.com.

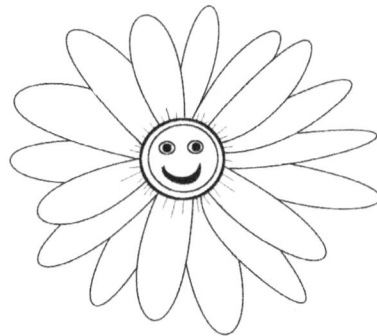

Made in the USA
Las Vegas, NV
20 February 2022